Item herba columbina in testiuo extinguit libidinem
Item mynthe contrita alijs cum succo veruene et pone
ad carne et eius efferuetur et spina tetigit exit men-
tis ad talia ita q cor tangentis emollit Item lapis
sulpteis portata in siniscis manu erectione virge
tollit Item testiculi galli cum sanguine suo supposita
lecto cubantid iacenti in eo venerem Item semen lactuce epositat spina et sedat desiderium coitus et pollucionem Item lapis topazius renat castitate erepit-
nut venerem Item succus iusiam testiculos undnige
tolore et tuolnee et libidinem extinguit Item lapis
ambrum portatus dat castitate. Item semen salic supe-
tid libidine extinguit Item coruce rute et agnus casti
sicceuit et pulneuenit et simul comedent tollent pollucionem. ¶ De duricia matricis et eius aspitate.
ffomentu aque decoccois maluie vel alice duricie
tollit. Item dug uncis et succus pnum nise et ungut
collid matricis post menstrua contracta matrice
relaxat Item lollid mixta thus al et contid simul
in vino vel aqua et fumet vel ungat clausa matrice apit et ad conceptio disponit ysaac. Item radix
elli elixata et fomentata dein dolorem tollit Item
succi nepte elist puocat Item empltum ex neptra
ante et retro prius torificata apo educit matrice
Item vinu decoccois origani puocat menstrua. Re-
oli li. j. collorintide ʒ. q. succo rute ʒ. iij. Absynthij p-
letru an ʒ. ij. et copia vit et c. ¶ De rtaricia vria
pacf eius succo marrubij bibita curat Item succus
ortice rubie cum seruisia bibita Item rasura eibor
bibita curat effit. Item crocus dissolutus in aqua
et potatus sanat statim. Succus camomille datus potin epatf fe cum aqua calida vrire pdel

# MEDIEVAL WOMAN'S GUIDE TO HEALTH

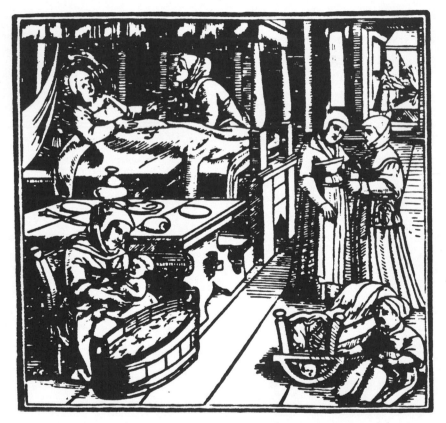

The lying-in-room in Jacob Rueff's *Ein schön lustig Trostbüchle*, 1554.

# MEDIEVAL WOMAN'S GUIDE TO HEALTH

*The First English Gynecological Handbook*

-¦-

*Middle English Text, with Introduction and
Modern English Translation by*

**Beryl Rowland**

-¦-

*The Kent State University Press*

This book has been published with the help of a grant from the Canadian Federation for the Humanities, using funds provided by the Social Sciences and Humanities Research Council of Canada.

Published in 1981 in the United States by
The Kent State University Press
Kent, Ohio 44242

Published in 1981 in Great Britain by
Croom Helm Limited
2-10 St. John's Road
London SW11

Library of Congress Catalog Card Number 80–82201
ISBN (U.S.) 0-87338-243-9
ISBN (U.K.) 0-7099-2216-7
Manufactured in the United States of America

**Library of Congress Cataloging in Publication Data**

English Trotula. English & English (Middle English)
    Medieval woman's guide to health.

    A Middle English treatise associated with Trotula;
edited from British Library ms. Sloane 2463.
    Bibliography: p.
    Includes index.
    1. Gynecology—Early works to 1800.  2.  Obstetrics—
Early works to 1800.  3.  Medicine, Medieval.  4.  English
language—Middle English, 1100-1500—Texts.  I.  Rowland,
Beryl.  II.  Trotula.  III.  British Museum. MSS.
(Sloane 2463)  IV.  Title. [DNLM: QZ 290 M489]
RG85.E53  1980          618          80-82201
ISBN 0-87338-243-9

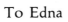
To Edna

# CONTENTS

# ILLUSTRATIONS

# NOTE ON THE ILLUSTRATIONS

The birth figures on pp. 124—33 were drawn from the originals in the manuscript Sloane 2463, ff.217–18v. by my sister, Edna G. Murphy. I wish to express my gratitude to her and also to: the Bodleian Library for permission to reproduce the illustration of a doctor attending the birth of Caesar in Jean Duchesne's translation of *de bello Gallico* in 1474 (MS. Douce 208, f. 1); the British Library for permission to reproduce the domestic scene in the early fifteenth-century *le livre et la vraye histoire du bon roy Alixandre* (MS. Roy 20, B XX, f.86v), and the illustration depicting the birth of septets in the fifteenth-century French romance *Le Chevalier au Cygne* (MS. Roy 15, E VI, f.273); the Royal Observatory, Edinburgh, for permission to reproduce illustrations of a doctor and patient from a fifteenth-century German astrological-medical manuscript (Cr. 4.6, f.84), and of midwife, mother, and infant from a fifteenth-century German miscellany (Cr. 8.101, f.34); the Bibliothèque de l'Arsenal, Paris, for permission to reproduce the illustration of the conception of a child from the second part of Jean Mansel's *Vita Christi* (MS. 5206, f.174); the Bibliothèque Royale Albert, Brussels, for permission to reproduce the illustrations on multiple births (MS. 3701–15, ff.27, 28v, 29). The two illustrations on pp. 17, 40 are taken from Rösslin's *Der Swangern Frawen und Hebammen Rosegarten*, 1513, and those on the frontispiece and p. 43 from Jacob Rueff, *Ein schön lüstig Trostbüchle*, 1554.

# FOREWORD

Very few books, scholarly or popular, about the theory and practice of medicine in medieval England are available; consequently, any new addition to the small corpus of such writings is welcome. This early fifteenth-century *Medieval Woman's Guide to Health*, a treatise on obstetrics and gynecology, is especially welcome because it antedates by about a century what had hitherto been considered the first work on this topic in English.

Of previous publications, most are editions of texts: first came George Henslow in 1894, who printed some extracts from *Medical Works of the Fourteenth Century*; Fritz Heinrich's *Ein mittelenglisches Medizinbuch* followed in 1896. Another typical *Leechbook or Collection of Recipes*, both scientific and folkloristic, appeared in 1934, edited by Warren R. Dawson (often quoted on account of its facing translation); a similar *Liber de Diversis Medicinis* was published shortly afterward (in 1938) by Margaret Sinclair Ogden for the Early English Text Society (OS 207). Professor Ogden also edited *The Cyrurgie of Guy de Chauliac* (OS 265), complementing the editions by Björn Wallner of other writings of this great surgeon. Two major treatises are available in the Early English Text Society: the original Middle English versions of *Lanfrank's Science of Cirurgia* (OS 102) and Arderne's *Treatises of Fistula in Ano* (OS 139). Dr. Charles Talbot of the Wellcome Institute for the History of Medicine has written the sole general survey, *Medicine in Medieval England* (1967), and with Professor E. A. Hammond, has compiled a bibliographical register of *The Medical Practitioners of Medieval England* (1965). Also to be noted are a few short but authoritative articles by such scholars as Dorothea Waley Singer and Eileen Power, and, since it relates directly to the topic of this volume, *Women Healers in Medieval Life and Literature* (1943) by Muriel Joy Hughes. All these works, however, are designed for the specialist with a good command of Middle English.

*Medieval Woman's Guide to Health* is of course directed to specialists in Middle English studies. But because of its subject matter, this volume will appeal in addition to a far larger class of nonspecialist readers, and for these the forbidding format of the typical scholarly edition with historical and linguistic apparatus, textual notes and glossary, has been discarded in favor of a simpler arrangement: an exploratory introduction on women healers in early medicine followed by the Middle English text along with—justification enough for publication—a facing translation. On account of the numerous technical terms, often much abbreviated, the text is difficult, and no doubt even Middle English specialists may find the translation helpful.

Manuscripts of Middle English medical texts have yet to be catalogued: no one knows what manuscripts are preserved, where they are located, or even what is in them. I have myself examined hundreds of medical treatises and collections of recipes, and many hundreds more which after inspection proved to contain no pertinent items. In 1970 I published in *Speculum* a preliminary survey of 350 Middle English medical manuscripts, but this figure is surely less than a quarter of the estimated total. Examining collections for texts of a certain treatise could easily continue for decades, and no assurance could be given that the search would ever be complete. With such personal experience in mind, and with the knowledge that a new project had been launched to catalogue *all* Middle English prose texts, I urged Professor Rowland not to look for further manuscripts of the "English Trotula" (as one manuscript rubricated it) beyond the twenty or so she had collected, but having decided on the superiority of Sloane MS. 2463, to publish that text without further delay. At least Middle English specialists would have a transcription, and the majority of readers unfamiliar with the language (but studying, say, the history of medicine or women's studies) would have a workable translation.

Physicians will find many curious sidelights, like the detailed instructions for surgical repairs, the traditions represented by herbal remedies, and the specific references to ancient authorities. But they will be chiefly interested in the contents of the thirteen chapters of the treatise, like the retention of the menses, irregular menstruation, prolapsis, hindrances to conception, pregnancy, difficult positions prior to childbirth, and the delivery of the child.

Although *Medieval Woman's Guide to Health* stakes no claim to a place in the feminist tradition, it nonetheless opens up, in the best pioneering tradition of women's studies, considerable new territory. Professor Rowland deftly identifies this treatise as a landmark in women's attempts to seek solace and assistance from other women; in the Prologue and throughout the whole treatise, its author in poignant and memorable passages stresses the importance of freeing women from their dependence on male doctors. The Prologue to the Latin version, it might be remarked, represents a response to the requirements of feminine modesty; the English version is a moving lament against one form of discrimination.

It is perhaps for this very reason that *Medieval Woman's Guide to Health* is less important in the history of medicine and more important in the history of women. Its author was intent on demystifying concepts of women's ailments, summarizing tried-and-true remedies rather than forwarding contemporary medical theory and speculation; the treatise was to serve as a handbook for midwives and perhaps for self-help. The later Middle Ages witnessed a plethora of how-to books, and this outpouring of handbooks on everything from husbandry to cookery to travel is recognized as a testimony to the developments of lay literacy and a growing bourgeois sophistication about technical expertise. Such books represented the aspirations of a people who looked to better and fuller lives through empirical knowledge. In this tradition, the "English Trotula" proves that English women of the late Middle Ages could express their female separateness and their own consciousness.

Many others besides physicians and feminists will obtain satisfaction from this volume. Social historians will note the assumption that ladies and nuns are particularly delicate creatures, requiring special medical care. Theologians may well be interested in the ethical and moral issues raised in discussions of curative therapy by sexual intercourse, and in the dilemma this remedy poses for nuns and unmarried women. Historians of science will see this text as an example of the late medieval dissemination of empirical knowledge. The vernacular handbooks preserved useful and workable advice, even though that advice was sometimes couched in the language of "humors" or justified by older theories. The Latin treatises, on the other hand, were too often anxious to exemplify the theoretical hypotheses of classical authorities in a medieval theological framework.

These are just some of the areas that can be probed from a variety of approaches. Professor Rowland's introduction is itself interdisciplinary, ranging widely through the accumulated learning of a dozen fields of endeavor, and bringing perceptive analysis to bear on a multitude of separate but interconnected problems. It is now up to the specialists in these other disciplines to pursue further the provocative issues Professor Rowland has raised and to carry our present knowledge of these matters beyond her initial analysis.

Rossell Hope Robbins
State University of New York at Albany

# PREFACE

The very earliest advisers on abortion demanded an agility from their patients that few women possess today. A Hippocratic treatise recommended that the woman on the sixth day of her pregnancy should perform a number of mighty leaps, making her heels touch her buttocks. After the seventh leap the "seed" would fall out of her with a clatter. Giving birth could be equally strenuous: to expel a reluctant fetus, the woman in labor was advised to run up and down steps, to fasten herself to a ladder which was then shaken violently, or to lie in bed with the foot-end raised high and then dropped.

In the Middle Ages, women lacked even this kind of consideration from the experts. Qualified physicians were largely concerned with male patients who, with the assurance of "satisfaction guaranteed or money back," often paid handsomely in advance for treatment. In times of the deadly bubonic plague especially, medical men such as Chaucer's "Doctour of Phisik," who "kepte that he wan in pestilence," ran a lucrative business, their patients being in no position to sue for malpractice. During these centuries there was no country doctor riding night or day through muddy lanes to deliver a child among the cows and pigs of the sooty hovel in which the mother lived. Even in the case of royalty, although the physician might hover in the antechamber wearing the splendid scarlet academic gown of the fully trained M.D., he did not inspect a woman's vital parts. Women's sicknesses were women's business. The European and Arabic medieval tradition was that while physicians might write some theoretical chapters on medical problems, they relied on women to carry out the actual operations and treatment. The most commonly repeated theoretical material, such as occurs in the Anglo-Saxon Leechdoms and other Old English fragments, was Hippocratic in origin and dealt with obstruction, sterility, miscarriage, retention of urine, hemorrhage, mental unbalance, enlargement of the womb, signs of pregnancy, formation of the fetus, prognostication of the sex of the child, and other matters. Medieval physicians were not concerned with the practical aspects of obstetrics, despite the fact that Soranus of Ephesus, who practiced in Rome during the reigns of Trajan and Hadrian, had written extensively on the subject. Even an eleventh-century work, purported to have been written for women by a woman called Trotula, contained no instructions on the actual delivery of the child, and *The Byrth of Mankynde*, translated from Eucharius Rösslin's *Rosegarten* (1513, and printed in London in 1540 and in an enlarged edition in 1545), is still occasionally regarded as the first obstetrical text to appear in English.

The manuscript which I publish here in its entirety for the first time preceded the publication of *The Byrth of Mankynde* by nearly one hundred years. A curious feature of the work is that although one copy of it is ascribed to Trotula, it contains material on obstetrics that appears to derive from Soranus. Preserved in the British Library, it is a handsome manuscript with capitals decorated in red, blue, and some gold leaf, and is evidently the work of a professional scribe. By 1563, it had passed into the hands of the Master of the Barbers' and Surgeons' Company—clearly not someone for whom the work was originally intended—and on his death it was purchased for forty-eight shillings and fourpence by one, John Feld. In 1875, Dr. J. H. Aveling, Physician to the Chelsea Hospital for Women, published a few pages of the manuscript. Himself a notable antifeminist, strongly opposed to allowing women into the medical profession, Aveling, ironically enough, claimed that by temperament women were especially unsuited to the practice of obstetrics. Yet this manuscript, which is specifically addressed to women, suggests that at one time women were the sole obstetricians. It also raises larger issues concerning the kinds of roles women formerly played in medicine.

Who the writer of the first English gynecological handbook was, we do not know. The professional scribe who made the copy, Sloane 2463, was almost certainly male, and for this reason I refer to "him" rather than "her." At the same time, I have kept in mind that the original treatise may have been written or translated from the Latin by a woman. The debt to the experience of women, whether such material was originally recorded orally or written down, is obvious throughout the work.

Such are the matters with which this present work is concerned. I should particularly like to thank Dr. Charles H. Talbot who has guided me throughout this study. His generous counsel and scholarly criticism have been invaluable. With the xvii

aid of a fellowship from the Canada Council, I have been able to
examine a number of primary texts at the British Library, the
Bodleian Library, the Wellcome Institute, the Library of the
Royal College of Surgeons, and the Academy of Medicine in
Toronto. These libraries, the Scott Library at York University,
and other libraries such as the Pontifical Institute of Mediaeval
Studies, the Warburg Institute, and the Huntington Library,
have been indefatigable in procuring special works for me.

There are other acknowledgements of a more personal
nature. I am grateful to my sister, Edna G. Murphy, who
prepared the illustrations for this book. I am also indebted to
Professors Sherman M. Kuhn, Margaret Jennings, OSJ, Rossell
Hope Robbins, Cyril Smetana, OSA, Dr. Gwyn Stuart Thomas,
A. D. Trapp, OSA, Margaret Whittaker, Pamela Gradon, Gail
McMurray Gibson, and my husband, Dr. E. Murray Rowland,
for opinions on specific points. Finally, as a Fellow of
McLaughlin College, I must express my gratitude to the Master,
Professor George Doxey, and to the Administrative Assistant
Molly Klein for their moral support, and to Rita Dallison and
Peggy Truman for their unfailingly competent and genial
secretarial assistance.

Beryl Rowland
McLaughlin College
York University
Toronto

# MEDIEVAL WOMAN'S GUIDE TO HEALTH

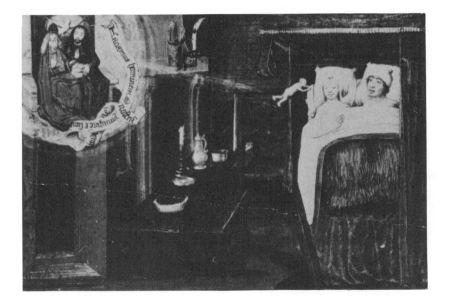

The Holy Trinity sends down a child on a ray of light to a couple lying in bed. The role of the Trinity in the creation of Adam and Christ is here extended to include a secular birth, with a scroll bearing witness to the significance of the scene: "Faciamus hominem ad imaginem et similtudinem nostram" (Arsenal MS. 5206, f. 174).

# INTRODUCTION

I n 1306, when Edward I of England and Philip the Fair of France were too busy consolidating their own kingdoms to think of conquering Jerusalem, lawyer Pierre Dubois, an enterprising political pamphleteer, put forward a scheme for recovering Western influence in the Holy Land. Let intelligent, good-looking women be trained as doctors, marry Eastern potentates, and use their talents and position to gain power. As a preparation, the women should be educated from the age of four or five in Latin, Greek, Hebrew, Arabic, medicine, and surgery.[1] Dubois's plan, though it was not accepted, is nevertheless an ingenious one. It refines those bedroom aspects of female espionage that can still blight promising political careers and crush aspirations to high office. More important, it suggests that medicine was one profession to which women had some entitlement, and it raises a question of interest today: to what extent did women, in fact, practice medicine in medieval times?

Women with some knowledge of the medical properties of plants, minerals, and parts of animals have existed in every century, in both fiction and fact. According to Homer's *Odyssey*, Helen of Troy learned the properties of drugs from Polydamna, in Egypt, "where everyone is a physician and acquainted with such lore beyond all mankind" (IV. 229). In the palace of Menelaus, she surreptitiously gave the guests a potent drug in their wine, and "who ever drank this mingled in a bowl, would not let one tear fall all day long, not even if his mother or father died, nor if his brother or dear son was slain before his eyes." According to Plutarch's biography of Mark Anthony, Cleopatra made daily experiments with various lethal drugs on criminals to discover which poison was the least painful in its operation. As the result of her observations, she concluded that asp poisoning, which she herself later used, was the "most eligible kind of death." In A.D. 54, the infamous Agrippina used Locusta, a woman druggist who had just been sentenced on a poisoning charge, to murder her husband, the Emperor Claudius. In Agrippina's view, the act was timely because Claudius had at last agreed to let Nero, her son by a former marriage, succeed him, instead of his own son. The poison was sprinkled on some exceptionally fine mushrooms, but owing, says Tacitus, to Claudius's natural sluggishness or intoxication and to a motion of his bowels, it was so slow in working that a feather tipped with a quicker acting toxin had to be rammed down his throat to hasten his death.[2]

Feminine skill in midwifery, which was to be vehemently challenged in the seventeenth, eighteenth, and nineteenth centuries, was, of course, recognized in early times, but in ancient Greece and Rome women seem to have practiced medicine on equal terms with men. Hyginus, the superintendent of the magnificent Palatine library under Augustus, tells of a woman called Agnodice, who disguised herself as a man in order to attend medical lectures in Athens. Subsequently, she became a widely respected gynecologist, and when her sex was disputed on account of her proficiency, she simply raised her tunic to show her femininity.[3] She was prosecuted for her medical activities.

In Rome much of the gynecological work appears to have been done by women. Some of these women were midwives (*obstetrices*), others were given full acknowledgment as doctors (*medicae*). Martial, in his epigram on Lydia, describes a situation in which a young woman tells her aged husband, with much regret, that intercourse is necessary to cure her hysteria. The husband acquiesces, and immediately, says Martial, the women doctors (*medicae*) depart and the men doctors take over. Josephus refers to an insurrectionist in Gamala as the son of a female physician.[4] Tablets on which women were described as *medicae* as distinct from *obstetrices* were set up in Italy, France, the Iberian peninsula, and elsewhere. In western Spain, for example, in the former Roman city of Merida, once famous for its magnificent granite bridge with eighty-one arches, its temples, and its theaters, a tombstone was erected by her husband to the incomparable wife (*uxori incomparabili*) and best doctor (*medicae optimae*),[5] Julia Saturnina, who had died at the age of forty-five. Among the Teutons, according to Tacitus, the practice of medicine was entirely in the hands of women.[6]

In the fifth century, Theodorus Priscianus dedicated the third book of a medical treatise to Salvina, addressing her as the gentle servant of his art.[7] In the sixth century, a Greek physician, Aetios of Amida, writing on women's diseases and childbearing in his *Tetrabiblon*, quoted extensively from one

Aspasia. Aspasia has been variously identified as the beautiful Phoenician mistress of Cyrus the Younger and of Artaxerxes, and as the Athenian courtesan who dominated Pericles. The dramatist Aristophanes even held her responsible for the Samian and Peloponnesian wars. Whoever she was, Aetios apparently regarded her as a remarkable gynecologist and obstetrician.[8] In the same century, at Poitiers, Queen Radegunde, wife of the homicidal Clotaire I, transformed her royal palace into a hospital for indigent women and went among the sick, washing them, and attending to their sores.[9]

In the eleventh century, from the flourishing medical school of Salerno in Italy, came Trotula, to whom was attributed an important treatise on the diseases of women and the care of children. Salerno's physicians referred to women practitioners and even to a certain *mulier Salernitana* who cured hemorrhoids with fig juice, but whether Trotula herself can be included in this catalogue of *medicae* is debatable. Trotula's work was known under various titles as *De passionibus mulierum curandarum, De aegritudinibus mulierum, De curis mulierum, Trotula major,* and *Trotula.* Sometimes works dealing with cosmetics and the care of the complexion, *De ornatu mulierum* and *Trotula minor,* were appended. In addition to entire manuscripts, certain chapters entitled *Practica domine Trote ad provocanda menstrua* and *Practica de secretis mulierum* were frequently copied, their popularity being due in part, in the opinion of one critic, to their "pornographic character."[10] *De passionibus mulierum curandarum,* first printed in 1544 at Strassburg, states in the preface the reason for the book:

> Since then women are by nature weaker than men it is reasonable that sicknesses more often abound in them especially around the organs involved in the work of nature. Since these organs happen to be in a retired location, women on account of modesty and the fragility and delicacy of the state of these parts dare not reveal the difficulties of their sicknesses to a male doctor. Wherefore I, pitying their misfortunes and at the instigation of a certain matron, began to study carefully the sicknesses which most frequently trouble the female sex.[11]

That Trotula was a woman and wrote the works ascribed to her was denied as early as 1566 by Caspar Wolff, who maintained in *Harmonia gynaeciorum,* the first part of an essay prefacing an encyclopedia of gynecology, that *De passionibus mulierum curandarum* was written by a Roman freedman of the Empress Julia named Eros or Erotes—"Erotis medici liberti Juliae, quem aliqui Trotulam inepte nominant in mulierum liber. . . ."[12] Wolff's contention seems tenuous, but Trotula's claims to authorship have never been satisfactorily established. Earlier in this century, such feminist medical historians as Mélanie Lipinska and Kate Campbell Hurd-Mead were convinced that she existed, and Elizabeth Mason-Hohl, in the preface to her translation of Trotula's work, stated that at Trotula's funeral in 1097, her casket was attended by a procession of mourners two miles long.[13]

However, the connotations of *trot*, already proverbial in the Middle Ages, are too suggestive to be ignored.[14] A *trot* was a *vieille*. She trotted for a living. Deprived of physical attractions by age, she had the wisdom of a sorceress, and in her business as procuress, she taught her protegées the tricks of the trade. *Besoing fait vieille troter* was an old French proverb. Old Trot was the stock joke of popular literature—the old woman who still wished to associate herself with sexual pleasures.[15] To the medieval misogynist, she was the repulsive creature that the promiscuous, proud, and desirable young woman inevitably became. "More than all of them I despise / The old woman [*la viele trot*] who is flirtatious, / When her breasts are withered," declared John Gower, Chaucer's contemporary, in his indictment of humanity, *Mirour de l'Omme* (ll. 899–901). As old as Ovid's Dipsas, *La Trotière* appears in all the major vernacular literature of the West and is defined as *"une femme de mauvaise vie."*[16]

Some of the recipes attributed to Trotula in the Latin text, such as "on the manner of tightening the vulva so that even a woman who has been seduced may appear a virgin" (xxxv) and "on adornment and whitening of the face" (lxi), are the same as those which the stereotyped *vieille* (*vekke, vecchia, vetula, annicula*) passed on to young women. Traditionally, as in the *Roman de la Rose*, the *vieille* gave instruction on feminine personal appearance, hygiene, eating, and drinking as part of her advice on how to ensnare men (ll. 13281 ff.). Although her own hideous appearance was a cure for the kind of love she had inspired as a young woman, she was knowledgeable in matters of contraception and abortion and had some repute as a midwife. Much to the horror of medieval moralists, she was even called *medica* and

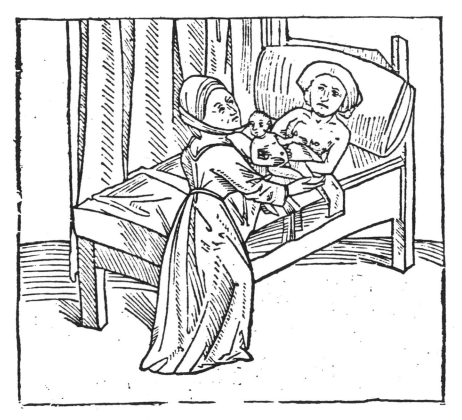

A successful birth.

thereby associated with an estimable profession.[17] Although
Cotgrave in his *Dictionarie of the French and English Tongues* in 1611
defined *trotiere* as "a raumpe, fisgig, fisking huswife, raunging
damsell, gadding or wandering flirt," usually she was old.
Gammer Gurton, in the early English comedy *Gammer Gurton's
Needle*, is called an "old trot," and the editor John S. Farmer, who
is better known for his dictionary of slang, glossed *trot* as "old
woman; usually in contempt, a drab, slut, strumpet."[18] A similar
implication is made by Shakespeare in *The Taming of the Shrew*: "an
old Trot, with ne'er a tooth in her head although she may have
as many diseases as two and fifty horses" (I. ii. 89). Sixty years
later Urquhart, translating Rabelais, described "an ugly old Trot

in the company" who "had the reputation of an expert she-physician."[19] The widespread use of the word and its association with expertise in feminine matters may explain why a medical compendium on women's diseases came to be ascribed to Trotula.

But if Trotula's authenticity remains in doubt, one of the more cautious scholars of the history of science and medicine has stated that a woman called Metrodora wrote a treatise in Greek on the diseases of the womb that "seems quite valuable" and is "probably the earliest extant medical treatise written by a woman."[20] It is in a single manuscript of the Laurentiana, Florence, entitled *Ek ton Metrodoras peri ton gunaikeion pathon tes metras*. As in the case of Agnodice, however, the designation seems almost too appropriate.

The name Trotula was associated with the medical school of Salerno, and in the fourteenth and fifteenth centuries women doctors did practice in the city.[21] Women do, in fact, seem to have been tolerated in medical practice as in no other profession. One reason for such tolerance is that caring for the sick was regarded as charity and came within the scope of those who were in orders, nuns as well as monks. By long tradition, the Church concerned itself with three kinds of institutions for the sick: (1) the monastic infirmary accommodating several physicians and sick monks, with special rooms for bloodletting and purging, and with a drug dispensary and herb garden nearby; (2) an institution mainly concerned with general charity but giving some medical aid; and (3) a hospice caring for the poor and elderly, but in which *cura aegrotantium*, even as applied to a leprosarium, involved providing food, clothing, and shelter rather than professional nursing or medical treatment.[22]

Medieval infirmaries, in general, appear to have been carefully organized and to have had recourse to expert advice in the monastic libraries. The library of the monastery of Christchurch, Canterbury, possessed more than two hundred titles of medical interest in its thirteenth- to fourteenth-century catalogue, and there were almost as many in the fifteenth-century catalogue of St. Augustine, the neighboring monastery, including works by Trotula, Galen, Hippocrates, Avicenna, Theophilus, and Dioscorides, as well as the popular *Regimen Sanitatis Salernitanum*. The smaller library of Dover Priory also contained nearly one hundred volumes on medicine, including *Trotula major*. [23]

The indications are that both nuns and monks, such as the Prior of Bermondsey referred to in the manuscript Sloane 2463, f. 200v, dispensed medical advice to female parishioners. In addition, there were secular lying-in hospitals for women. The Close Rolls in 1344 and 1353 state that should a mother die in childbed in the hospitals of St. Mary-without-Bishopsgate and St. Bartholomew, the child should be cared for until the age of seven. At Holy Trinity, Salisbury, "lying-in women" were to be cared for until they had been delivered, recovered, and churched. St. Thomas at Canterbury looked after women in childbirth, as well as pilgrims en route for Rome. Another famous refuge with women in attendance was provided for women at St. Thomas, Southwark, by the London mercer Richard Whittington, who died childless in 1423. According to William Gregory, one of Whittington's successors to the London Mayoralty:

> The noble merchant Richard Whittington made a new Chamber with eight beds for young women who had done amiss in the hope of good amendment and he commanded that all the things that occurred in that room should be kept entirely secret under pain of loss of livelihood. For he would not shame any young woman in any way because it might prove a hindrance to her marriage.[24]

Among the women of the Church was an abbess, St. Hildegard of Bingen, who tackled all branches of medical science known in the twelfth century, as well as philosophy and theology. Her *Causae et Curae*[25] is a mini-encyclopedia defining the human condition in both moral and physical terms, beginning with the creation of the world and the fall of Lucifer and concluding with the causes of fever which, Hildegard claimed, were slothfulness and various kinds of self-indulgence. Her contemporary biographers, Godfrid and Theodoric, while regarding her ability as miraculous, seemed to have considered her medical activities within the scope of a woman, although admittedly her cures appear to have been effected by psychological rather than medical means.[26] Her fame, apparently inspired more by her healing powers than by her writings, reached far outside her small nunnery on the Rhine. Even the humble speaker in the fourteenth-century Middle English *Pierce the Ploughmans Crede* exhorts his readers to listen to Hildegard ("Herkne opon Hyldegare").[27]

In secular life also, women of necessity treated a variety of ailments. Qualified physicians were not likely to be found in rural districts, and the lady of the manor or the wise woman of the village was expected to cope with medical emergencies. Recipes were handed down from mother to daughter, even in royal households. Often repeated is the story that Queen Philippa (1314–69), wife of Edward III of England, was sent by her mother a copy of a book from the School of Salerno and some plants of the herb rosemary.[28]

Numerous medieval romances and histories describe situations in which women were expected to give medical treatment and did so. In Boccaccio's *Decameron*, in the story of the Third Day, Giletta, who is explicitly called *Donna Medica*, takes charge of the patients when her physician father, Gerard de Narbonne, dies. Her greatest triumph is in curing the King of France of a fistula. Women apparently dressed wounds successfully, especially those in the leg and shoulder, using herbs as both plasters and potions. It would seem from such poems as the German romance *Tristan* by Gottfried von Strassburg (1210) that gentlewomen on occasion went onto the battlefield, carrying their medicine bags with them. In the same poem, Blancheflor, who is secretly in love with Rivalin, contrives to visit him by posing as an *arzatinne*, a woman doctor;[29] the lady in the romance of Bevis of Hampton knows physic and surgery because she studied both subjects in Armenia: "While she was in Ermonie / Both fysik and surgirie / She hadde lerned of meisters grete."[30] Some manuscripts provide illustrations of women at their work. The history of Tobit, in an illuminated manuscript of the *Historia scholastica* at the British Library (MS Royal 15 D.I), shows an old man in the background, lying blind and sick on his couch. In the foreground his wife prepares a medicament for him. With an air of composure and professional competence, she sits before a large fireplace, keeping one hand on the page of her manual of instructions, while with the other she uses a ladle to stir the contents of a pot. With justice, the indefatigable medievalist Thomas Wright remarked in his *Womankind in Western Europe* in 1869, "The question of allowing women to practice as doctors has been a subject of great discussion of late, but in and before the feudal period it [the practice of medicine] was regarded as one of the natural duties of the sex."[31]

The extent to which women were permitted to carry out

these "natural duties" varied. In Spain and the south of Italy, where the universities and the medical faculties were under governmental and not ecclesiastical jurisdiction, women were able to obtain a license to practice. In Germany also, women practiced medicine and were given the title of *ärztin*. In Frankfurt alone, between 1394 and 1500, more than a dozen women doctors are recorded. Some of them were Jewish, for, despite stringent Church prohibitions, Jewish physicians were in demand in northern Europe throughout the medieval period. They were knowledgeable because they had access to Arabic-Greek medical works in Hebrew translation, and their reputation was enhanced by the traditional concept of the Jew as sorcerer.[32] Although in 1494, at Frankfurt, a Jewish *ärztin* was forbidden to practice either general medicine or gynecology, Jewish women doctors continue to be registered, some of them being designated oculists (*augenärztin*). Usually the woman doctor appears to have been treated with some respect and was not regarded as a quack (*heilkünstlerin*).

On the other hand, in France, in 1311, the medical faculty of the University of Paris took steps to prevent the practice of medicine by unlicensed persons, declaring that a statute which, it was said, had existed many years, must be enforced. The chartularies contain references to an official opposition to women doctors, and, significantly, the first practitioner to whom the faculty of the University of Paris objected was a woman. In 1312, Clarice de Rothomago was arrested at the instance of the Dean for the unlawful practice of medicine and was excommunicated. She appealed, but her sentence was reconfirmed and her husband was excommunicated as well.[33] Ten years later, Jacqueline Felicie de Almania, aged about thirty, was excommunicated for the same reason. Her case was heard before John of Paris, with many witnesses testifying that she had cured them of fevers, ulcers, and other maladies. In her defense, Jacqueline maintained that the prohibition, made in 1220, referred only to ignorant women ("totaliter ignora artis medicine et non litterata") —a group from which she was excluded because of her training and knowledge. The argument she made is one that prefaces nearly all medical works intended for the use of women:

It was more fitting that a wise woman, experienced in the art of medicine, should visit another woman, to examine

her and to inquire into the hidden secrets of her being, than
that a man should do this. For a man is not permitted to do
these things, nor to investigate or feel women's hands,
breasts, stomach, feet, etc. On the contrary, a man ought
to avoid the secrets of women and fly from their intimate
association as much as he can. Also a woman would let
herself die rather than reveal the secrets of her infirmity to
a man, because of the virtue of the female sex and because
of the shame which she would endure by revealing them.[34]

Jacqueline was again found guilty, and other women practitioners—Jeanne Conversa, Margarita de Ypre, and Belota
Judea—were also excommunicated and prohibited from engag-
ing in medical work.

In 1352, King John of France forbade anyone of *either sex* to
give medical treatment except under certain conditions.
Practitioners had either to be masters or licentiates in the
science of medicine of a university, or to be acting under the
direction of a master of the University of Paris, or otherwise
approved by the faculty of medicine. In 1390, Charles VI issued
a further ordinance. However, despite the threat of expulsion,
imprisonment, and even death, women in Dijon, Lyons,
Rheims, and many other places continued to practice medicine.

In England the records testify that women did practice
medicine, notwithstanding increasing opposition. Only five
names are cited, and for the three about whom details are
available, professional life seems to have presented problems.
Pernell de Rasyn, practicing on the Devonshire coast at
Sidmouth, was involved in an unpleasant situation of the kind
that, so it is currently alleged, one physician in every four faces
during the course of his career: she was sued for malpractice.
The complaint was that she and her husband Thomas, also a
physician, caused the death of a local miller through their
medical incompetence. The case was settled by a royal pardon in
1350. Earlier in the same century, a leech (healer) known as
Margery of Hales, in Worcestershire, found herself in trouble
with the lord of the manor for various offenses such as causing
property damage by allowing her cow to stray and gathering
nuts and chopping firewood on the manorial preserves. She was
fined, and on one occasion she was thrown into a river to
determine whether she was a witch. Another leech, Johanna of
Westminster, who received payment from the abbey infirmary

during 1406–7 for medicines, was probably the same Joan who wanted a license to practice physic "without hindrance or disturbance from all folk who despise her by reason of her said art" and petitioned Henry IV to this effect. There is no record of the king granting her request. Nothing is known of the two remaining women physicians: Agnes, *medica* of Stanground, Huntingdonshire, and Katherine, *la surgiene* of London, both practicing in the last quarter of the thirteenth century.[35]

In 1421, physicians petitioned Parliament to limit the practice of *fysyk* to university-trained graduates and to declare that "no woman use the practyse of fysyk."[36] Their request was granted two years later. Nevertheless, the proliferation of manuscripts suggests that women continued to practice medicine, and in the medieval vocabulary, a "Fysycian or leche" was "Mann or woman: Medicus, medica."[37] Although the illiterate old wise woman of the rural community with her herbs, folklore, midwifery, and "witchcraft" was undoubtedly active, as she had been up to that century, there were, in addition, women physicians who read manuals and sought to practice obstetrics and preventive medicine. Some of these manuals were in Latin, but at this time a remarkable change occurred: whole treatises, written by laymen for laymen, appeared in the vernacular. The phenomenon had social implications. As Rossell Hope Robbins observes, "the difference in language separated the relatively few university-trained physicians like Chaucer's 'Doctor of Phisik' from the un-Latined others, specifically the on-the-job-trained surgeon, barber-surgeon, apothecary, apprentice, cunning man, wise woman, lay sister in a convent, and midwife."[38]

As far as women were concerned, probably comparatively few could read and write with any fluency. The education of women was limited because of many factors, including that of early marriage, which was legal at the age of twelve. The elderly martinet Philip of Navarre, in his treatise on *The Four Ages of Man*, thought that even a rich girl should not be taught to read or write unless she were to become a nun; if she were educated, he argued, she might read foolish letters sent by admirers who would never have dared to convey their messages verbally (i. 25). Literacy in the modern sense would not have been general among women, and the writer of the vernacular manuscript was addressing himself to the exceptional rather than the usual woman. Let "euery woman lettrid . . . Reede to other vnlettrid"[39] is his advice.

The increase in translations may also have been partly due to the fact that even in religious houses not all women knew Latin. The translator and paraphraser of the Register of Charters of the Benedictine nunnery of Godstow, near Oxford, written for the use of nuns in the time of Dame Alice Henley (elected abbess 1445–51), explains that he undertook to write in English because a lack of understanding of the Latin text and a dearth of learned men to advise the nuns could cause "grete hurt and hyndraunce." Similarly, even the offices used in their religious observances were translated for the sisters of the Brigittine monastery of Sion, at Isleworth, because some of them were unable to read Latin.[40] In the case of medical vernacular manuscripts, the possibility exists that some of them were written in commercial scriptoria for speculative sale. Rossell Hope Robbins observes that the repetition of similar recipes, often in similar order, is strongly suggestive of this practice.[41]

Because these vernacular manuscripts were mostly translations, the craft of medicine they presented was essentially the same as that in the Latin treatises. First would come the prognosis, the astrological calculations of the possibility of effecting a cure and the best time for treatment. Chaucer credits his well-qualified "Doctour of Phisik" with being particularly skilled in this aspect of the healing art. Indeed, the professionally trained doctor often carried prognosticatory tables and equipment necessary for accurate zodiacal calculations. One such aid was the volvelle, consisting of several revolving vellum discs and a revolving pointer, which showed the days of the month, the zodiacal signs, the symbols of the months, and the days of the solar and lunar year. The computing was complicated and does not appear in such vernacular manuscripts as Sloane 2463, even though various writers including Hildegard had urged parents to note the time of conception in order to facilitate astrological calculations.[42]

Next followed diagnosis, derived chiefly, by ancient tradition, from an inspection of the urine. Eighteen different significant colors are specified in the chapter on uroscopy in the Breslau Codex, and the importance of uroscopy was constantly emphasized. "If the change in pulse indicates that the individual is sick," states a somewhat sophisticated treatise, De Cautelis Medicorum, attributed to the thirteenth-century Spanish physician Arnaldus de Villanova, "the kind of disease is still better indicated by the urine. . . . While you look at the urine for a long time, you pay attention to its color, substance and quantity and to its contents, from the diversity of which you will diagnose the different kinds of disease, as is taught in the Treatise on Urines."[43] Linacre, physician to Henry VIII, tried to put an end to the abuse of uroscopy by formulating a statute that prevented physicians from diagnosing and prescribing from a mere inspection of the urine, often without even seeing the patient. The practice was, of course, related to the theory that discoloration of the urine was caused by the excretion of superfluous humors. In diagnosis, therefore, the physician attached great importance to the disposition of the humors, being convinced that any disease was caused by the presence of an excess of some one quality in the body.

Finally, there was the treatment of the disease, mainly by use of herbs, parts of animals, minerals, metals in potions, fumigations or baths, bloodletting, and cupping. Some of these treatises were in verse, possibly as an aid to memorizing. A fourteenth-century poem on bloodletting gives advice similar to that which appears in Sloane 2463: "A woman xal in the hanmes blede / for stoping of hire floures at nede."[44]

These manuscripts were numerous because in late fourteenth- and fifteenth-century England there were hundreds of unlicensed practitioners serving the medical needs of anyone in their local areas who could afford treatment. Indeed, when physicians petitioned for a "closed shop" in 1411, only about sixty of them were university trained, although many empiricists, women as well as men, undoubtedly worked on cases that demanded a knowledge not only of "fisyk" but of surgery. Such practitioners were harshly criticized by notable physicians. In his treatise on medical science, *Inventarium seu collectorium cyrurgie*, which the famous surgeon and resident physician of the papal household at Avignon completed in 1363, Guy de Chauliac complained of quacks who relied on the saints to cure all sickness, believing that the Lord had given the sickness and would take it away when it pleased him. A fifteenth-century Middle English translation of his work classifies women with *ydeotis* (the unlearned) or *foles* (fools).[45] The famous physician John Arderne scornfully recorded the unsuccessful treatment of a patient who "was under the cure of a lady by halfe a yere."[46] Arnaldus de Villanova, in the proem to the third book of the *Breuiarium Practice*, observed, "In this book I intend, God being my helper, to treat of those sicknesses which particularly concern women, and as women are in general venemous animals I shall follow it up with a treatise on the bite of venemous animals."[47] Even more scathing were the observations of John Mirfeld, an unbeneficed priest who lived in a priory of Augustinian Canons and was apparently associated with St. Bartholomew's Hospital in the late fourteenth and early fifteenth centuries. In a chapter entitled "De Medicis et eorum Medicinis" in his *Floriarium Bartholomei*, he denounced the "worthless and presumptuous women" who "usurp this profession to themselves and abuse it; who, possessing neither natural ability nor professional knowledge, make the greatest possible mistakes (thanks to their stupidity) and very often kill their patients." Mirfeld hoped that even "the poor and unlearned without many books" might benefit from his Latin medical compilation *Breviarium Bartholomei*, but he wrote solely for men and provided some strange recipes, including one for making gunpowder.[48]

Despite the contempt for women both as physicians and patients evinced by these writers, there was some awareness that women required special medical treatment which might best be undertaken by women practitioners. The manuscript from which the text is published here, Sloane 2463, belongs to the group of Middle English treatises on childbirth and women's diseases that is directed to women. Some such treatises may have been written by women, and more than one such manuscript exhorts every learned woman to read it to those who are unlearned, and to help and advise them in their sicknesses, without showing their diseases to man. The reason for providing the manuscript in the vernacular is often stated. A Douce manuscript explains, "Because whomen of oure tonge donne bettyr rede and undyrstande thys langage than eny other and euery whoman lettyrde rede hit to other unlettyrd and help hem and conceyle hem in her maledyes, withowtyn shewyng here dysese to man, i have thys drauyn and wryttyn in englysh."[49] But whether the compiler of Sloane 2463 was a woman, we do not know. Nor can we be certain of the writer's profession. When medical opinion is quoted, the expression "physicians sayne" does not necessarily indicate that the writer was a physician. Allusions that seem autobiographical must be treated with caution. Another contemporary medical manuscript ends with a statement implying that the writer, despite his clear, regular hand, is some kind of apprentice medical practitioner: "Now in this fyne of the particle y shal make an end . . . for thys in my masterys time and myne I haue. That well preued and cured and helyd many a pacyent, thanked by god of hys grace sendyng to that is the heyghest and the beste leche. Amen."[50] Yet even this seemingly personal statement was probably copied, for a similar conclusion appears elsewhere: "For this in my masteris tyme and myne haue welle preued and cured and heled many a pacient, thanked be god of his grace tendyng to that is the heighest and the best leeche."[51] When John Mirfeld alludes to his "master" in his medical compilation he is merely quoting from well-known medieval textbooks. In our manuscript, the lavish decoration of the first initial suggests that this copy may have been made for a noble lady, possibly acting as instructress on her estate. The hand is that of a professional scribe, and the work may well be one of those collections of medical recipes written in commercial scriptoria.

If an author is addressing a treatise to women, he or she usually makes the intention clear at the outset, expressing dismay at the thought of the work falling into men's hands. If that happens, a man must read it for one reason only—to help women. Women are, however, naturally modest and should be treated by other women, as our writer observes:

> Because there are many women who have numerous diverse illnesses—some of them almost fatal—and because they are also ashamed to reveal and tell their distress to any man, I therefore intend to write about curing their illnesses, praying to merciful God to send me grace to write truly to His satisfaction and to the assistance of all women. For charity calls for this: that everyone should work to help his brothers and sisters according to the grace that he has received of God. And although women have various maladies and more terrible sicknesses than any man knows, as I said, they are ashamed for fear of reproof in times to come and of exposure by discourteous men who love women only for physical pleasure and for evil gratification. And if women are sick such men despise them and fail to realize how much sickness women have before they bring them into this world. And so, to assist women, I intend to write of how to help their secret maladies so that one woman may aid another in her illness and not divulge her secrets to such discourteous men.

The writer also urges men to take a different attitude to women's illnesses:

> But nevertheless, whoever he be that offends a woman because of the malady that she has by God's command, commits a great sin; for he despises not only women but God who sends such sickness in their best interests. And therefore no one should despise another for the disease that God sends but should have compassion and help if he can.

The attitude expressed here, already traditional, is to be repeated through the centuries. As we have seen, it was given as a defense of women practicing medicine in medieval France, and even in the eighteenth century Daniel le Clerc maintained that the reason women had been so active in medicine was that most women had difficulty in disclosing certain secret illnesses to men.[52] Similarly, the writer of the preface to the 1718 edition of *Culpepper's Compleat and Experienc'd Midwife*, which purported to be a translation of "Aristotle's most elaborate treatise on the subject," expressed the hope that he might make the midwife a skillful physician, because he knew that "such is the Pudor and Bashfulness of many young women who happen to be affected with those Distempers that are common to their Sex, that they had rather die than discover them to a Doctor."[53] At the same time, Dr. John Maubray, in his preface to *The Female Physician containing all the Diseases incident to that Sex, in Virgins, Wives and Widows . . . to which is added the Whole Art of New Improv'd Midwifery*, declared that women had been finally taught "to lay aside all *childish Bashfulness* and *imaginary Modesty*, in order to secure their *Own* and their *Children's* safety, by inviting the *Assistance* of both SEXES."[54] But Maubray was proselytizing for "man-midwives," and was anxious to strengthen the long-standing attack on women amateur practitioners. Except among the poor, the business of the accoucheur was too lucrative to be passed over by male physicians.

The antifeminist remark of Dr. Walter Harris, physician to William and Mary in the latter part of the seventeenth century, is typical: he refers to "those charitable ladies, who living in Country Places, at a great distance from any good Physician, kindly practise Physick among their poor Neighbours, and give *Cordials* for all sorts of Complaints, or to delight the ignorant with Medicines that seem agreeable to their Palates. . . . And

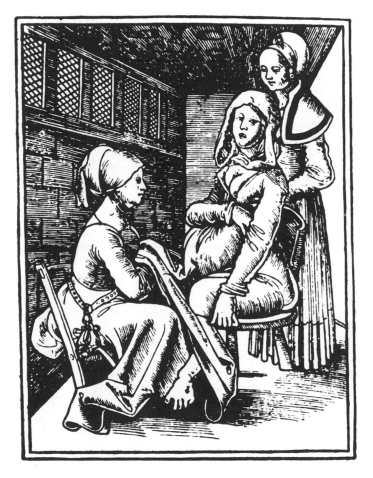

The birth-room in Eucharius Rösslin's *Der Swangern Frawen und Hebammen Rosegarten*, 1513.

yet it is a Matter of Doubt with some of the best Physicians, whether of those who have not died a violent Death, *more have perished by Diseases or by Cordials*."[55] Yet his own book purporting to deal with diseases of infancy, avoids any reference to obstetrics, even though it deals with pica in somewhat exaggerated terms ("there have been some, whose appetites have been so enormously depraved, that no eatable could satisfy their longing, but what was taken from some fleshy or callous Part of the human Body"), and with the nursing of children.

Printed works on gynecology and obstetrics were few and

were designed for the kind of practitioners whom Harris castigated. The earliest was *Das Frauen Buchlein*, 1500, attributed to Ortollf von Bayerland; the most important was a work published in 1513 by Eucharius Rösslin, a city physician at Frankfurt-am-Main. His book, *Der Swangern Frawen und Hebammen Rosegarten* ("A Rose Garden for Pregnant Women and Midwives"), was instantly popular and had three editions in the same year. It was reprinted ten times by 1568 and translated into Dutch, Czech, French, Danish, Latin, and English. The first English version was translated in 1540 from the Latin version *De Partu Hominis* by "a certaine studious and diligent clerke" named Richard Jonas. Three years earlier, Jane Seymour had died of puerperal fever after the birth of Edward VI, and this work was dedicated to Henry VIII's new wife, Catherine Howard. Jonas's translation was enlarged by Thomas Raynalde in 1545, and it is this work, entitled *The Byrth of Mankynde, otherwyse named the womans book*, which became well known in England. It was reprinted in 1552 and lived on until 1676, the new editions of 1560, 1564(?), 1565, 1593 (?), 1598, 1604, 1613, 1626, 1634, 1654, and 1676 containing few alterations or additions. The prologue to the first edition suggests, as did our Sloane manuscript, that the writer was aware of existing prejudice:

> For consyderynge the manyfolde / daylye / and imminente daungeorus and parelles / the which all maner of women of what estate or degre so euer they be in theyr labor do sustayne and abyde: yea many tymes with parell of theyr lyfe / of the whiche there be to many examples nedelesse here to be rehersed. I thought it shulde be a very charitable and laudable dede: yea and thankefullye to be accepted of all honorable and other honest matrons / yf This lyttell treatyse so frutefull and profytable for the same purpose were made Englysh / so that by that meanes it might be redde and understande of them all / for as touchynge mydwyfes / as there by many of them ryght expert / diligent / wyse / circumspecte / and tender about suche busynesse: so be there agayne manye mo ful yndyscreate / unreasonable / chorleshe / & farre to seke in suche thynges / the whiche sholde chieflye helpe and socoure the good women in theyr most paynefull labor and thronges.[56]

19

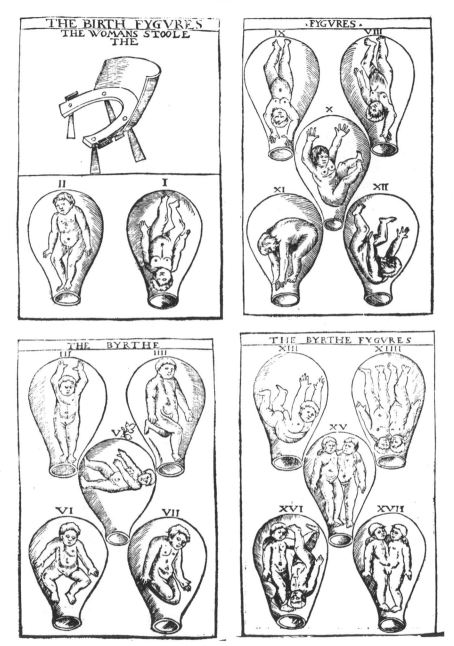

The birth stool and the birth figures from Thomas Raynalde, *The Byrth of Mankynde*, 1552 ed.

In edition after edition, the writer expresses the fear that, should the book fall into "light merchants hands," it might be used "to the discredit of women, that men might hereby conceive a certain . . . abhorrance toward a woman." At the same time, he urges women readers not to be offended with what "is spoken of the body." By the late eighteenth century the theory and practice described in this text was not valued very highly, although reservations about bringing "women's matters" before the public were still expressed. In the nineteenth century Dr. J. H. Aveling, despite his antiquarian interests, dismissed *The Byrth of Mankynde* as "full of the grossest blunders," and his own *History of our Midwives and of their Ignorance and Incompetence* shows that he failed to understand the problems of the time and the primitive state of medical practice as a whole.[57] *The Byrth of Mankynde*, like Sloane 2463, was a compendium of the knowledge available at that time and repeated many of the recipes and descriptions to be found in our manuscript.

Such material, in turn, derives from earlier writers. Theories on gynecology and fetal physiology, the nature of women's complaints, antedate Hippocrates. Cited in subsequent treatises for many centuries were ideas ascribed to Hippocrates, such as the etiology of the mole (Lat. *mola*), signs of death of a fetus, remedies for the prolapse of the uterus, the belief that the right side was connected with a male infant and the left with a female, tests for female fertility by means of fumigation, and various signs of pregnancy. The first extensive work of the Christian era on the subject, that of Celsus, was not discovered, however, until the latter half of the fifteenth century and therefore had little influence in medieval times. Pliny in his *Historia Naturalis* gave some gynecological data and description of the medical use of herbs. About A.D. 77, his contemporary Dioscorides wrote a pharmacological compendium that had an influence extending beyond the Renaissance. For diseases of women, he advised internal medication, application of poultices, unguents, fumigations, baths, and he dealt with most of the subjects treated in our manuscript.

Of the medical writers who followed in what has been regarded as the most brilliant period in the history of ancient medicine, extending to the end of the second century, the most authoritative, as subsequent writings on gynecology and obstetrics attest, was Soranus. Soranus made accurate observations on the nature of the uterus and the changes experienced in pregnancy, and was a keen clinical observer. He described and prescribed for cases of difficult labor and miscarriage, and correctly observed that the most favorable time for interrupting pregnancy was in the third month. He has been credited with being the originator of podalic version, and he described the birth stool, an item used centuries earlier by the Egyptians and Israelites. His *Gynecology* represented the body of knowledge collected by the early second century and was the main authority after Hippocrates. His Greek text remained only in one badly corrupted manuscript, and after its discovery by Conrad Gesner in the Augsburg library, it was even given a wrong attribution by Caspar Wolff when published in 1566. Nevertheless, during the Middle Ages, Soranus appears to have been an almost legendary figure. In the catalogue of the library of Christchurch, Canterbury, which contained his work, he was described as physician under the patronage of Queen Cleopatra, a name persistently associated with gynecology.[58] His writings had a precarious history and are probably far from complete as we have them now.[59] They were transmitted in the Middle Ages through various Latin and Greek paraphrases, the most important and best known being a Latin abridgment by Muscio, a writer whose identity is uncertain. Muscio's work exists in a number of manuscripts. Originating about A.D. 500, the abridgment was translated into Greek in Byzantine times, and the earliest extant manuscript is the Codex Bruxellensis dating from the ninth century.

Of those who succeeded Soranus, Galen (b. A.D. 129), though influential and, indeed, regarded by many as the supreme medical authority for the centuries following Hippocrates, was not an obstetrician, and his teachings on the anatomy of sex organs were no improvement over Soranus, except in his description of the Fallopian tubes. His knowledge was derived from the dissection of female genitalia in animals, and he considered the human uterus bicornate. Among those who made Soranus more widely available was Theodorus Priscianus. Predating Muscio by about a century, and writing in Greek and then translating, he based the third book of his *Euporista* on Soranus. Caelius Aurelianus in the next century produced a Latin version of the *Gynecology*, ranging from paraphrase to almost literal translation. The Byzantine writers also drew heavily on Soranus: the earliest, Oribasios (325–405), dealt with a variety of women's complaints and with pregnancy and immediate postpartum care. Aetios of Amida (502–75), court physician to Justinian, Emperor of Byzantium, besides tackling the same subjects, dealt in detail with difficult deliveries (xxii). He put head presentation first and stated that

> of the remaining positions, that which is less suspicious [dangerous] is a foot presentation [breech] particularly if the fetus comes out with a hand extended over each thigh. The fetus which comes out by one foot while the other foot is retained [in the uterus] or those with both feet doubled up and leaning on either side of the vulva [uterus], need straightening as do those who have outstretched hands.[60]

His material on childbirth is very close to Soranus (IV. 3), from whom he obviously drew. Paulos of Aegina (625–90), while essentially a surgeon, was an obstetrical consultant, and his text was accessible to the Arabian authors and highly valued. The Arabian authors themselves took most of their gynecology from previous Greek and Latin authorities, and while some of them referred to a vaginal speculum, custom decreed that they should leave the practical aspects of obstetrics, including the management of difficult childbirth, to women. Of these writers, Rhazes (b.865), Haly Abbas (d. 994), Albucasis (936–1013), and Avicenna (980–1037) were held in high esteem in the West. Rhazes taught that head presentation required no manual interference, but in all other presentations the hand was to be inserted in the womb to correct the presentation. Like the scribe of Sloane 2463, he advised anointing the genitals with oil to stimulate labor pains. Albucasis's text, which was printed by Wolff, was a standard text in the Middle Ages even though, in the Arabic tradition, medieval physicians were apparently not trained to deal with childbirth and were dependent on women to carry out the actual operations and treatment.

Instruction on the delivery of the child is often omitted by encyclopedists and medieval writers. Famous as the Salernitan school was in the eleventh century, its medical writings repeated prescriptions from Hippocrates and Galen for curing women's diseases. Trotula's best-known work, *De passionibus mulierum curandarum*, contains chapters on menstrual disorders, sterility, pruritus, signs of pregnancy, difficult parturition, infant feeding, choice of a nurse, problems of women after childbirth, and a variety of other matters, but little about childbirth itself. Indeed, nearly half her text is concerned with material seldom mentioned in Sloane 2463 and other similar manuscripts, such as severe coughing of children, foul-smelling sweat, ailments of the eyes, vaginal problems arising from coition, rupture of the vulva, pain of the vulva, women urinating in bed, methods of tightening the vulva to give the appearance of virginity, recipes for women who abstain from intercourse, for fat women, cures for dysentery, lice, eczema, cancer, skin irritations, swelling of a man's testicles and penis, small pimples in children, foulness of breath, worms of hands and feet, deafness of ears, inflammation of the tonsils, toothache, fistula, roughness of hands, instructions for facial makeup, including treatments to eliminate wrinkles, freckles, and red spots, and descriptions of a water of life or distilled elixir, and recipes for the preservation of sight.

The reason that writers neglected the subject of presentation at birth and the different ways of dealing with it cannot be established with certainty. Whether their avoidance of the subject was deliberate is doubtful. They freely disseminated the Graeco-Roman world's techniques of contraception, amplified by some concoctions from Rhazes and Avicenna, not because they were promoting contraceptive practice but because they were prepared to treat fully a topic for which they had pertinent information.[61] On the practical aspects of childbirth they presumably did not have accessible data. Arnaldus de Villanova has a chapter on difficult births: he finds two natural modes of birth, headling and footling; in other cases he recommends manipulation by the midwife to effect normal delivery.[62] On the other hand, Bartholomew the Englishman's encyclopedia, popular as it appears to have been in the fourteenth and fifteenth centuries, has only one chapter "de obstetrice," and this chapter is concerned with child-rearing rather than with midwifery.[63] In the middle of the same century, Vincent de Beauvais in his *Speculum* dealt with pregnancy, sterility, and involuntary abortion but referred to childbirth only briefly, stating that it was facilitated if the woman was made to sneeze ("Sicut Hippocras ait").[64]

The limitations of professional advice on childbirth are especially apparent in Guy de Chauliac's *Inventarium*, the Latin treatise which, as noted earlier, was copied and translated into English in the same period as Sloane 2463. "A newe borne childe," stated the famous surgeon, "goth out proprely vpon his hede, the face turned toward the erthe. All other goyinge oute forsothe is vnkyndely and harde." The woman should be encouraged to sneeze by the use of pepper or milkwort, and the plant agrimony should be fastened to the patient's thigh to hasten the birth "as wise men sayne." A dead fetus could be detected by various signs: contraction of the nipples, lack of movement in the womb, coldness, foulness of breath, sunken eyes, lack of feeling in the lips and the whole face. In such cases, he recommended the use of fomentations, pessaries, abortive medicines such as dried beaver gland, myrrh, and rue. If these failed, the midwife should use a speculum, open the womb as wide as possible, and then draw the fetus out with hooks either whole or in pieces. If the woman was dead and the fetus alive, the law forbade the woman to be buried until the child was delivered. In which case, he instructed, the midwife was to open the woman "with a razor on the left side (for that part provides better access than the right because of the liver), and put in thy fingers, and draw out the child. Julius Caesar, forsooth, was drawn out in this way. . . . " The surgeon's remarks indicate that he was relegating the day-to-day operations to women and was not concerned with the finer details. His attitude is made clear when he refers to multiple births: "Childbirth is also made difficult because of many children; sometimes there are two, and according to Avicenna five or more, and according to Albucasis more than seven, even ten, so he says. And because the matter requires the attention of women, there is no point in giving much consideration to it."[65]

By going into detail concerning the various forms of unnatural birth and the remedies, our manuscript is therefore dealing with material not always treated by the encyclopedists and practitioners of the time. The later printed books did not improve upon the work until Paré's midwifery was translated into English in 1612. Even in the next two centuries the birth instructions closely resembled those in Sloane 2463. Philip Barrough, for example, repeated them in *The Method of Physick* printed in London in 1653. A century later, William Smellie, in a work on midwifery that, following a long tradition, he attributed to Aristotle, gave similar instructions.

But if the obstetrical details in Sloane 2463 are not found in the textbooks of the famous medieval physicians and surgeons, they were nevertheless in circulation in English by the fifteenth century. Very similar redactions can be found in MS 129a.i.5 at

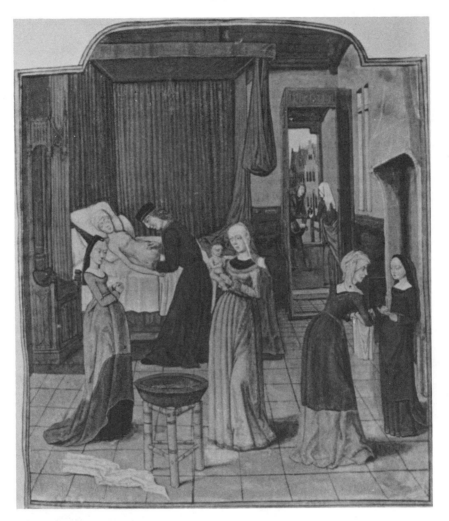

A male doctor attends the birth of Caesar (MS. Douce 208, f. 1).

the Royal College of Surgeons and in Sloane 249, from the John Wooton collection of medical treatises. There are also manuscripts in which part of the above traditional material appears, such as Sloane 5, ff. 158–73, BM Royal 18A, VI, ff. 35–54, BM Addit. 12195, ff. 157–85. Ultimately, much of the material in these redactions, apart from the details concerning childbirth, can be traced to texts of such writers as Roger de Baron, Gilbertus Anglicus, Arnaldus de Villanova, Albucasis, and others, whose writings on women's ailments contain chapters very similar to those in these vernacular texts, usually in the same order:

> On the Retention of the Menses
> On the Immoderate Flow of the Menses
> On the Suffocation of the Womb
> On the Precipitation of the Womb
> On the Excoriation of the Womb
> On the Wind in the Womb
> On the Aposteme of the Womb
> On the Impediment to Conception
> On Difficult Childbirth
> On the Secundine
> On the Passion of the Womb
> On the Inflation of the Breasts
> On the Swellings of the Legs in Pregnant Women.[66]

The peculiarly English character of Sloane 2463 is evinced by certain references (that also occur in Sloane 249) from London or the Home Counties. Powdered roots of dragaunce (dragon-wort) and leaves of march (parsley) in "good ale" cured the Baron of Surcester's wife[67] of an almost fatal hemorrhage of the womb (p. 81); for excessive menstruation a recipe of burnt hartshorn and eggshell powdered in soup, sauce, or drink proved very effective in Cheapside (p. 81); a herbal recipe for dropsy cured a woman whose life was despaired of by London doctors (p. 111); a certain recipe of the Prior of Bermondsey saved a woman almost dead from a hemorrhage of the womb (p. 77); in Essex, which had a very active tanning industry at Colchester,[68] a woman was cured of the flux when she sat in a bath of herbs boiled in tanner's juice, up to her navel, "as long as sche may endure" (p. 85). In addition, there are allusions to persons whose recipes proved efficacious, Richard Marche (p. 161) and Lightfoot (p. 163), both with common English surnames,[69] but otherwise unidentifiable, and to an Edmund, "Edmund magister" (p. 156) or "Edmonds prest" (p. 164n), who presumably was St. Edmund of Abingdon (1180–1240), Archbishop of Canterbury. Edmund was the first Oxford master to be officially canonized, and in the opinion of his biographers his fame for healing exceeded that of St. Thomas à Becket. Matthew of Paris and others record how the saint nursed a sick pupil for five weeks and effected many miraculous cures. At his interment at Pontigny, clubs had to be used to disperse the crowd. A mob rushed to kiss some part of the body or bier, and according to one eyewitness, "contact therewith seemed to bring health to everyone."[70] Other biographers declared that miracles continued in all parts of the world where the name of Blessed Edmund was invoked.[71] That our manuscript should refer to him is therefore not surprising. Various relics of the saint were brought to England, and his name was associated with healing for many centuries.

The general procedure in the Sloane manuscript is to state the complaint, describe symptoms, the reasons for the complaint, and the cure. This approach to the subject is one which continues in many of the printed treatises, even in the compendiums attributed to Culpepper published in the seventeenth and eighteenth centuries. The divisions are those made by qualified practitioners for their own use, as well as by the writers of popular handbooks. Even in 1746, Dr. D. D. Fitzgerald, in his handwritten Latin treatise, *Tractatus de morbis mulierum*, retained the traditional rubrics and arranged each chapter under specific headings: *Descriptio et Definatio, Differentia, Causae, Symptomata, Diagnosis, Prognosis, Curatio.*[72] At times, however, the text of the Sloane manuscript becomes a jumble of recipes, which the writer seems to have copied somewhat indiscriminately. Latin recipes, including many with unusual case endings and constructions, are mixed with English recipes at random, and the treatise ends with a medley of recipes having to do with conception, the stone, colic, and palsy. In addition, moralistic attitudes intrude upon the general pattern: "for certainly it is better for man or woman to have the greatest physical illness while they live than to be healed through a deed of lechery or any other deed against God's commands" (p. 91).

The remedies in Sloane 2463 are drawn from many sources. The principal recipes are potions, consisting of herbs, parts of trees, fruit, minerals, parts of animals, including turtledoves or eels burned alive (pp. 81–83), and many of these ingredients are boiled in special liquids such as wine or vinegar. Suppositories, made chiefly of herbs, are to be tied by a thread to the thigh to prevent displacement (p. 69); cupping, bleeding, and herbal baths are frequently recommended. Like Trotula, the writer advises vinegar for swollen legs, but further suggests that one should take what lies under the smith's trough, beneath the grinding stone, dry it, make a powder of it, and mix it with the vinegar and anoint the place. Such a recipe is also good for "man's feet" and for "legs that travel by the roads" (p. 153). Whereas Soranus was interested in the mental and physical well-being of his patients and advised pregnant women to "promenade, exercise the voice and read aloud with modulations, take active exercise in the form of dancing, punching the leather bag, playing with a ball, and by means of massage" (I. 49), our writer is not concerned with such matters and does not mention exercise or general diet. On one occasion, for stone in the womb, he advises that the woman should be induced to sneeze and then made angry before being given a suppository (p. 145). He is enthusiastic about fumigations, for which he recommends an *embote* (p. 102), a syringe or douche, in order to introduce curative fumes or liquids into the body, and he accepts the belief, stemming from Hippocrates, that the womb was connected with the digestive tract and ultimately with the mouth and nose. Not surprisingly, therefore, to cure the suffocation of the womb (hysteria), he advises the application of foul-smelling things to the nose and aromatics to the vagina:

> let the patient smell stinking things that are exceptionally odorous, such as burnt felt, dog's hair, goat's hair, or a horse's bone set alight and then extinguished, or hartshorn, old shoes, burnt feathers, a wick, moistened in oil, ingnited and then extinguished, a woollen rag, or a live smoking coal. . . . And from the navel down to the privy member anoint her with fragrant things such as ointments and oils, and make a fumigation underneath of pleasant, sweet-smelling things and draw the matter down from the heart. [pp. 91–93]

Soranus had contemptuously rejected such procedures:

> The majority of the ancients and almost all followers of the other sects have made use of ill-smelling odors (such as burnt hair, extinguished lamp wicks, charred deer's horn, burnt wool, burnt flock, skins and rags, castoreum with which they anoint the nose and ears, pitch, cedar resin, bitumen, squashed bedbugs, and all substances which are supposed to have an oppressive smell) in the opinion that the uterus flees from evil smells. Wherefore they have also fumigated with fragrant substances from below, and have approved of suppositories of spikenard and storax, so that

the uterus fleeing the first-mentioned odors but pursuing the last-mentioned, might move from the upper to the lower parts. . . . The uterus does not issue forth like a wild animal from the lair, delighted by fragrant odors and fleeing bad odors; rather it is drawn because of the stricture caused by the inflammation. [III. 29]

Nevertheless, the traditional ideas persisted in the writings of Aetios, Trotula, and others, and when our writer deals with the falling of the womb, he naturally recommends the reverse procedure, applying evil-smelling things to the womb and sweet-smelling items to the nose. Even in the eighteenth century, after the theory of the uterine origin of nervous diseases had been challenged, the practices described by our author were still recommended: "Apply sweet scent to her nose, civet, galbanum, styrax, calamitis, wood of aloes. . . . And let her lay stinking things to the womb, such as Assa-Foedita, Oil of Amber, or the Smoak of her own hair being burnt; for this is a certain truth, that the womb flees from all stinking, and to all sweet things."[73]

Today no one would deny that psychological states may be affected by the menstrual cycle, and the long-continued use of the traditional remedy may be due to some vague realization of the connection. The persistence of the belief that the womb was sensitive to smells and moved accordingly probably accounts for the widespread use of smelling-bottles up to this century. These small bottles, often made of cut glass, once resided in every household and even accompanied the afternoon tea tray. Containing carbonate of ammonia and colored yellow, green, or pink, the salts were most frequently applied to the noses of fainting or hysterical young women. As a child in an age when juvenile amusements were limited, the present writer remembers the thrill of unstopping the mysterious little bottle on the dressing table and sniffing its pungent contents. Some druggists still stock such bottles.

On the nature of generation, our writer implies that the "seed" is in both man and woman. He not only refers to women retaining their seed but, in the case of the mola, he suggests that the disorder may occur if the woman's own seed is unfertilized. There were several views on generation. According to Aristotle, the seminal fluid for generation was produced by man alone, the female menses providing the passive matter on which the male seed worked.[74] This view was general in the Roman world and was asserted by Jerome and Augustine,[75] as well as by later writers such as the "cursed monk" Constantine (b. 1087), who specialized in aphrodisiacs.[76] Soranus attached even less importance to the female role. He likened the act of procreation to "sowing extraneous seed upon the land for the purpose of bringing forth fruit" (I. 36). Muslim physicians of the ninth and tenth centuries, on the other hand, referred to both male and female seeds, the one having a kind of coagulative power and the other having a receptive capacity for coagulation. Our writer does not define his interpretation of seed but it would seem that his view is similar to that expressed by Avicenna.[77]

Occasionally, statements in our manuscript are a divergence from the usual. For example, pica is not specifically connected with pregnancy. When the writer says that a woman in a certain condition may have a desire to eat coal, rinds, or shells, he appears to associate pica with failure to menstruate (p. 63). Yet most works stated that pica was a sign of pregnancy. The description of the mola in the womb differs from that of Soranus and Aetios in several respects. Our manuscript recommends herbal baths, anointing the lower part of the body, wrapping the patient in a hot double sheet, fumigating the private parts with sweet-smelling things, applying with a feather a vaginal douche of bull's gall and other herbs mixed, while the woman lies with her head low and her "taylende" high (p. 142). Then, in the most drastic remedy, which necessitates winding two towels round the patient's middle and applying a stick either side, tourniquet fashion, a mola appears to be a fetus, whereas most authorities regarded it as a tumor.

Elsewhere the copious alternate recipes suggest that originally they were culled from several manuscripts. On folio 225v (p. 152 ff.), after the recipes on swelling legs, there is an extended note on *ad menstrua provocanda*. It continues in Latin, derived, one would assume, from another manuscript. On folio 229v (p. 166), with a new paragraph, the style changes; and whereas the writer has previously used either the imperative or the jussive subjunctive, he now speaks first-person plural and continues thus until folio 230 (p. 168), when, in citing a fertility recipe similar to Trotula's, he uses the imperative again. Nor does the work adhere to the original plan. Folios 194v–195 (pp. 58–61) set out ten disorders of the womb and indicate that a chapter will be devoted to each. The scheme breaks down by the fifth chapter, which deals with "wind" in the womb (p. 105) instead of ulceration, and there is no rubric for the sixth chapter. The rubrics appear to have been inserted separately, and it would seem that the scribe forgot to put a rubric in the space on folio 211v (p. 109) before "dropsy." Chapter 7 deals with the "rawness" of the womb rather than with the swelling, and Chapter 8 treats the inflammation of the womb, which was announced as the sixth topic. Chapter 9 gives as its subject the aching of the womb, Chapter 10 grievances in childbearing, and Chapter 11 the withholding of the secundine. There are also two additional chapters: Chapter 12 which gives recipes for making a woman conceive, and Chapter 13 which deals with excessive bleeding after childbirth (p. 147) and subsequently provides recipes for restraining sexual intercourse (p. 157), jaundice (p. 159), swelling of the testicles (p. 161), and other matters.

On a subject closely associated with midwifery for centuries, the practice of magic, our writer says little. Yet contemporary literature reflects considerable popular belief in a variety of supernatural aids. In one fourteenth-century manuscript, among four Latin charms given to facilitate childbirth is the beginning of the Athanasian creed, "quicunque vult," which must be said three times over the woman in labor.[78] In vernacular manuscripts, charms often appeared untranslated, especially, it seems, in connection with childbirth—"O infans, siue viuus, siue mortuus, exi foras, quia Christus te uocat ad lucem!" ("O infant, whether living or dead, come forth because Christ calls you to the light!").[79] In 1481, Agnes Marshall, alias Saunder, was arraigned in a York visitation for using incantations in childbirth,[80] and with the advent of the Reformation "charms, sorcery, enchantments, invocations, circles, witchcrafts, soothsaying, or any like crafts or imaginations invented by the devil, and specially in time of women's travail" were frequently condemned. In 1538, Nicholas Shaxton, Bishop of Salisbury, advised every curate to charge midwives not to use "girdles, purses, measures of our Lady or such other superstitious things" in order to persuade a woman in childbirth that her labor would be easier as a result.[81] Similarly, in an inquiry in Kent in 1576, people were asked "whether there be any among you that use sorcery, or witchcraft, or that be suspected of the same, and whether any use charms or unlawful prayers, or invocations in Latin or otherwise, and, namely, midwives in the time of woman's travail of child, and whether any do resort to any such help or counsel, and what be their names."[82] The earliest example of the midwives' oath, dating from 1567, includes the promise to refrain from using sorcery or enchantments during labor. The only ritual permitted during labor was to baptize the child when death seemed imminent. Then either the midwife or one of the parents should say: "*Creatura Dei, ego te baptizo in nomine Patris, & Filii, & Spiritus sancti*" ("Creature of God, I baptize you in the name of the Father, Son, and Holy Ghost"). Such baptism might occur when the child was half born, with only the head and neck visible, or if the mother died and the midwife ripped her up to try and save the child: "And yef the wommon thenne dye / For to undo hyre wyth a knyf / And for to saue the chyldes lyf, / And hye that hyt crystened be."[83] No "rose or damask water, or water made of any confection of mixture" was to be used.[84]

Our writer makes little use of such superstitions. Although he treats of the secundine, he has no reference to the caul, despite the fact that superstitions regarding its magical properties were ancient and persistent.[85] Even the pseudoscientific predetermination of the sex of the unborn child, a tradition inherited from classical medicine that continued to be disseminated in the late seventeenth century, is not included. He has only two magical remedies to assist parturition: a precious stone and a girdle. Soranus had no faith in amulets apart from their possible psychological benefit to a credulous patient (III. 42). He did, however, recommend that a girdle of linen be worn until the eighth month and then discarded in order that the weight of the child might assist in bringing on labor at the proper time (I. 56). This girdle was employed for strictly medical purposes.

The kind of girdle to which our writer refers is one credited with supernatural powers. Trotula had advised wearing such a girdle (xvii), and in England childbirth girdles of various materials were in use from the time of the Druids until the nineteenth century, often remaining in the same family for many generations. Edward the Confessor gave the girdle of the Blessed Virgin to the Cathedral of St. Peter in Westminster, and it was carefully guarded by the sacristan. When Henry III led an expedition to Gascony in 1242, his wife Eleanor accompanied him, and she sent to St. Peter's for the girdle when she was in childbirth.[86] There is, however, no record of Eleanor having a child in 1246, the date given in the record, so one must assume that either the date was 1244, when her daughter Beatrice was born, or that the girdle proved ineffective. A contemporary of our scribe condemned the superstition at the beginning of *Pierce the Ploughmans Crede*, where he accused the Carmelite friars of making women think that a girdle from the  Virgin's dress assisted childbirth: "& maken wymmen to wenen / that the lace of oure ladie smok / lighteth hem of children."[87] Nevertheless, in 1536, the convent of Bruton was reported to possess "our Lady's girdle of Bruton, red silk, which is a solemn relic, sent to women travailing which shall not miscarry *in partu*," and another girdle, reputed to have belonged to Mary Magdalene, "sent also with great reverence to women travailing."[88] According to Sir Walter Scott, in an early witchcraft trial, Bessie Dunlop claimed that her familiar, one Thomas Reid, a soldier killed at the battle of Pinkie in 1547, gave her "a lace . . . out of his own hand which, tied round women in childbirth, had the power of helping their delivery."[89] In the Middle Ages, even manuscripts in roll form were used as birth girdles.[90]

Trotula's *De passionibus mulierum curandarum* had specified that the girdle was to be of snakeskin, a skin which a snake had sloughed off (xvii), but our writer recommends hart's skin (p. 139). In the same passage, Trotula also recommended a precious stone that would shorten the pangs of childbirth, *aetites*, the eaglestone. This stone has had a long history in obstetrics. It was supposed to prevent abortion and facilitate delivery if applied at the correct time. Dioscorides, Plutarch, and others believed that the eaglestone actually pulled out the unborn child and retained its power of traction long after the birth.[91] The Talmud recommended its use.[92] In the sixteenth century, a physician reported that a woman suffered a fatal prolapse of the uterus because a large eaglestone was not removed from her immediately after her delivery.[93] In the eighteenth century, the eaglestone was still being recommended along with other magical objects:

> The stone aetites held to the Priveties is of extraordinary Virtues, and instantly draws away both Child and After-birthen, but great Care must be taken to remove it presently, or it will draw forth the womb and all. . . . There are many other things that Physicians affirm are good in this Case: among which are an Ass's or Horse's Hoof hung near the Privities: A piece of red coral hung

near the said place: A loadstone helps much, held in the Woman's left hand; the skin which a Snake hath cast off, girt about the middle next to the skin.[94]

The procedure, according to Trotula, was to tie the stone to the thigh; in addition, a magnet held in the woman's right hand was considered to be efficacious (xv).

Our writer in the Sloane manuscript refers not to the eagle-stone, nor to the magnet, but to "*isapis*," no doubt a metathesis for "*iaspis*." Jasper amulets to facilitate childbirth date from the Graeco-Egyptian period.[95] Such amulets were also thought to increase lactation. On one ancient stone is carved the representation of a parturient woman seated in a delivery chair. According to the medieval lapidary, jasper "helpeth a woman in bering of children & deleverance." In the opinion of Albertus Magnus, the stone prevented conception, aided childbirth and kept the wearer from "licentiousness."[96] St. Hildegard of Bingen in the eleventh century recommended that the pregnant woman should have jasper in her hand for a full nine months in order to ward off malevolent spirits:

> And when the woman bears a child from that hour when she conceived it until she delivers, through all the days of her childbearing, let her have a jasper in her hand, so that the evil spirits of the air can do so much the less harm to the child meanwhile, because the tongue of the ancient serpent extends itself to the sweat of the infant emerging from the mother's womb, and he lies in wait for both mother and infant at that time.[97]

Petrus Hispanus maintained that the jasper would expel a dead fetus, and the same claim for the stone is made by our author (p. 206). The stone continued to be employed as an amulet during the sixteenth and seventeenth centuries, and is said to have been used in Greece even toward the end of the last century.[98] Also in fairly common use were topaz and amber which our writer recommends in a Latin recipe for restraining coitus. Less usual is his revelation that "lapis sulpicis" held in the left hand suppresses an erection (p. 156).

Another example of our writer's use of ancient ideas is the pregnancy test. It is a test that can be traced back to Egyptian papyri, and it turns up as the Galenic test for fertility.[99] Wheat or bran was put in two pots. The man watered one pot daily with his urine, the woman the other. According to a medical treatise that repeats the test: "That which grows first is the most fruitful, and if one grows not at all that party is naturally barren."[100] The writer of our manuscript uses a part of this ancient recipe for his fertility test (p. 169) but confuses it with another, as does *De passionibus mulierum curandarum*. Trotula's advice is as follows:

> If the woman or the man be sterile you will ascertain it by this method: take two jars and into each put bran. Into one of them put the urine of the man and into the other put the urine of the woman and let the jars be left for nine or ten days. If the barrenness be from a defect of the woman you will find many worms and the bran foul in her jar. On the other hand you will have similar evidence from the other urine if the barrenness be through a defect of the man. But if you have observed such signs in neither urine, neither will be the cause of the barrenness and it is possible to help them to conceive by the use of medicines. [xi]

Our writer follows the Latin Trotula fairly closely here, as well as in recommendations on how to produce a male child. In a recipe given by Pliny and others,[101] Trotula states that the man is to take the womb and vulva of a hare, dry it and pulverize it, blend it with wine, and drink it. The woman is to do the same with the testicles of the hare and to cohabit with her husband at the end of her menstrual period. Our writer advises both husband and wife to take a hare's womb and vulva and drink them in wine if they desire a male child. Should the woman desire a female child, she is to "dry the testicles of a hare, and at the end of her menstrual period make a powder of it, drink it at bedtime, and then go to play with her mate" (p. 169). Testicles of a pig are recommended for similar purposes.

The reason for recommending parts of the hare and the boar to promote fecundity is not hard to find. The ancient belief that to acquire certain qualities one should eat parts of animals believed to possess those qualities persisted even in the medical textbooks of the eighteenth century. The fertility tests themselves had an equally long life.

Although the theological implications of medical practice are not considered in the text, two references to abortion (pp. 97, 135) require some explanation in the light of modern controversy. In particular, the statement that "whan the woman is feble and the chyld may noght comyn out, then it is better that

the chylde be slayne than the moder of the child also dye" seems
to be counter to the relatively hard anti-abortion line, popularly
believed to express he traditional attitude of the Church, which
was advanced by the Holy Office as late as the end of the last
century and solemnly promulgated by Pope Pius XI in his en-
cyclical *Casti Connubi* (1930).[102] Of course abortion, especially
therapeutic abortion performed for the purpose of saving a
mother's life, was known and practiced by Greek and Roman
physicians, but by the first and second centuries A.D. abortion
was regarded as a social evil.[103] Several patristic writers denounced any type of direct abortion as being contrary to the
divine precept "Thou shalt not kill."[104]

The question raised was: at what point could the fetus be
regarded as "human"? According to Artistotle, the fetus became
human forty days after conception if it was male, ninety days
after conception if it was female. The prescription in Leviticus
12:1–5, that a woman must spend forty-five days of purification
if she has given birth to a boy and eighty days if she has given
birth to a girl, seems to imply a similar view. Among the Church
Fathers, divergent theories arose from discrepancies in the two
versions of Exodus 21:22. According to the Hebrew text, if a
man accidentally caused an abortion, life was given for life only
if the mother died; the death of the fetus was not treated like the
killing of an adult human being. In the Septuagint version, the
death penalty was prescribed if the embryo was "formed." The
prevailing Christian view seems to have followed the Septuagint in distinguishing between an unformed and formed
stage. Ensoulment was generally thought to occur at conception, but in his commentary on Exodus 21:80, Augustine argued
that "if the embryo is still unformed, but yet in some way
ensouled while unformed . . . the law does not provide that
the act pertains to homicide, because still there cannot be said to
be a live soul in a body that lacks sensation, if it is in flesh not yet
formed and thus not yet endowed with senses." The doctrine of
delayed hominization, taking Aristotle's prescription as the
norm, was extended by Aquinas, Gratian, and other scholastic
commentators and glossators into distinctions between formed
and unformed fetuses, with a concomitant lessening of moral
gravity in cases of the abortion of the unformed fetus.[105] Even
some strict anti-abortionists, such as Tertullian, approved of
therapeutic abortion: "Sometimes by cruel necessity, while yet
in the womb an infant is put to death, when lying awry in the

orifice of the womb he impedes parturition and would kill his mother were he not to die himself."[106] Soranus raised the moral issues:

> A controversy has arisen. For one party banishes abortives, citing the testimony of Hippocrates who says: "I will give no one an abortive"; moreover, because it is the specific task of medicine to guard and preserve what has been engendered by nature. The other party prescribes abortives, but with discrimination, that is, they do not prescribe them when a person wishes to destroy the embryo because of adultery or out of consideration for youthful beauty; but only to prevent subsequent danger in parturition if the uterus is small . . . or if some similar difficulty is involved. [I. 60]

In his recommendations for abortion, however, he prescribes for the "woman who intends to have an abortion," and he does not emphasize medical reasons.

Such an attitude would have been unacceptable in medieval times, when the Church's attitude toward abortion and contraception became more rigid. In the tenth century, Regino of Prum, listing the questions to be asked by the bishop on his pastoral visitation, stated, "If someone to satisfy his lust or in deliberate hatred does something to a man or woman so that no children be born of him or her, or gives them to drink, so that he cannot generate or she conceive, let it be held as homicide."[107] This text became canon law as the decretal *Si aliquis* in 1237. Although Henry de Bracton, chancellor of Exeter Cathedral, in his well-known treatise *The Laws and Customs of England*, completed in 1256, treated of abortion per se, when the effects of canon law were felt, abortion and contraception were grouped together, as an anonymous writer of the lawbook *Fleta* indicates:

> One is rightly a homicide who has pressed on a pregnant woman or has given her poison or struck her to produce an abortion or to prevent her from conceiving, if the fetus was already formed and ensouled, and similarly he who has given or received poison with this intention of preventing generation or conception.[108]

The common theological attitude would no doubt be that expressed by Chaucer's Parson or, even more explicitly, in

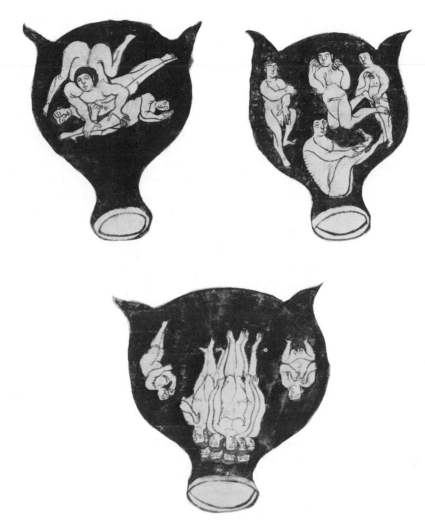

Fetus preparing to emerge from the womb, as illustrated in a tenth-century Muscio text.

another Middle English text: "For the slaying of children before they are christened, inducing abortion and destruction of offspring by medicine, is most sinful."[109] In Sloane 2463, however, therapeutic abortion seems to be considered sufficient justification in itself for adopting an attitude and recommendations contrary to those usually attributed to the Church.

In dealing with the delivery of the child and the problems that may arise, Sloane 2463 provides illustrations showing the fetus in various positions in the womb. These birth figures and the accompanying descriptions are the most remarkable feature of our manuscript. The birth figures are shown in a number of manuscripts,[110] and scholars usually assume that they derive from Soranus's *Gynecology*. There appears to have been a place for them in the text and, in the opinion of one scholar, the one extant, badly corrupted manuscript of the fifteenth century contains a reference to them.[111] Muscio included the illustrations, and his *Gynaecia* seems to have circulated widely in the Middle Ages, even turning up in a fifteenth-century Latin manuscript of John of Arderne's *De Arte Phisicale et de Cirurgia* in the Royal Library at Stockholm.[112] In the illustrations in the Muscio manuscripts, the uterus containing the fetus looks like a Florentine flask. Soranus had indeed compared the uterus to a cupping glass, and the flask is the usual representation of the womb in medieval and early printed texts.

Despite the alleged common source, however, the illustrations vary. In the case of multiple births, for example, the Codex Hafniensis, which represents the womb as a circle with a Florentine flask inside it, includes one set of twins, and they are descending feet first. The Codex Palatinus has two sets, the first showing twins descending feet first, the second showing one child presenting with the feet and the other with the head. The Codex Bruxellensis, in addition to showing triplets and quadruplets all presenting abnormally, displays nine well-developed, overweight homunculi bunched together at the mouth of the womb, ready to go out head first, while their two siblings squat patiently on either side, obviously resigned to a long wait.

None of the birth-figure illustrations displays any knowledge of the true nature of the embryo.[113] Although the fetus varies from manuscript to manuscript, it is always matured far beyond the prenatal stage, and in many instances looks like an adult, with fully formed genitalia. The variety in the drawings suggests that whereas compilers of bestiaries sometimes borrowed transfers from a scriptorium for their illustrations of elephants, lions, and other animals, the writers of gynecological treatises drew freely on their imaginations. Rösslin's illustrations show the most determined attempt to turn the fetus into an infant, a two-year-old of cherubic proportions, with dimpled cheeks, full abdomen, and fat legs.

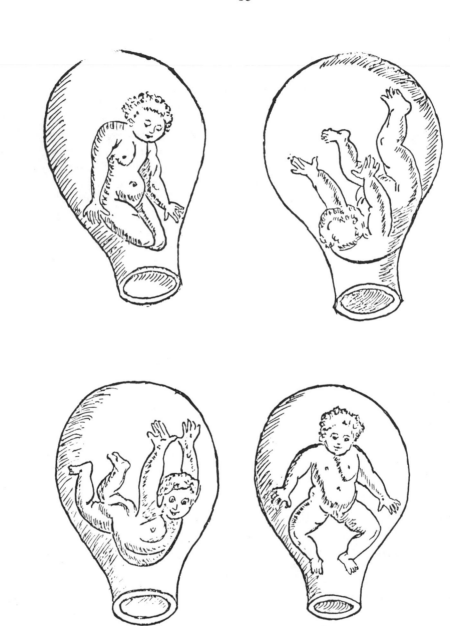

Various birth figures from Eucharius Rösslin's *Der Swangern Frawen und Hebammen Rosegarten*, 1513.

In our manuscript the art work is spectacular. The flask has become a sphere, and the first four birth figures which are numbered *i* in the left-hand margin in ink, stretch out like rose-pink balloons, one-third from the top of folio 217. The infants are drawn in black line and are colored a light flesh pink against the deeper pink background representing the uterus. Each infant is blessed with a mop of yellow hair outlined in black and looking rather like a shower cap or badly fitting wig. The other birth figures, which are in sets of four on ff. 217v, 218r, 218v, are similarly decorated and are numbered in the margins, *ij, iij, iiij*. The birth figures also appear in Sloane MS 249 and in the Royal College of Surgeons MS 129a.i.5. The birth figures in Sloane 249 resemble those in Sloane 2463, and display a pink circle as the womb. MS 129a.i.5, at the Royal College of Surgeons, on the other hand, is distinctive in that it shows a black infant, his eyes and mouth outlined in white, descending through a bubble of dark red plasma to a green half-moon at the base.

In Sloane 2463 all the illustrations deal with unnatural presentation, and the accompanying instructions inform the reader that the chief duty of the attendant in the case of a child presenting unnaturally is to push the child back into the vagina and try to rearrange it. In general, the recommendations appear to be traditional. Despite the span of centuries, Soranus and Gilbertus Anglicus gave substantially the same instructions, which are repeated here: correct malpositions manually and use ancillary measures such as hot baths, poultices, inunctions, fumigations, and applications of various herbs. There is, however, no reference to the "birth-stool," and whereas a contemporary English medical treatise, which also contains the birth figures, shows a woman in labor pulling on a cord fixed to a beam above the bed,[114] our scribe does not allude to the practice.

Vincent de Beauvais suggested that foot presentation was an acceptable alternative to head presentation.[115] Such a view is rare. Like Soranus, our writer regards head presentation with arms alongside the legs the only "normal" presentation, as it had been almost invariably since Hippocrates. Natural birth, says our writer, occurs when "the child comes out in twenty pangs or within those twenty, and the child comes the way it should: first the head, and afterward the neck, and with the arms, shoulders, and other members properly as it should" (p. 123). The twenty pangs (*throwes*) presumably mean twenty contractions of the uterus, implying a precipitous delivery, probably taking half an hour.[116]

Our writer describes sixteen ways of unnatural presentation and gives advice on how they are to be rectified. The descriptions are accompanied by illustrations, and the first is clearly a face presentation—"when the child's head appears as it were head first and the rest of the child remains inside the womb." Here the writer advises using hot herbal oils. The midwife is to anoint the birth canal, probably with the purpose of making the cervix open faster. This manual enlargement of the uterus, or *accouchement forcé*, is an ancient practice still known to gynecologists. The second presentation is "when the child comes with his feet jointly together and the midwife can never bring the child forth when he comes down like this." Here is a footling presentation with the legs flexed, coming out before full dilation has occurred. The advice is to push the child up again into the vagina (presumably to keep the child warm). The third unnatural manner is if "the child's head be so huge and so great that it cannot come forth." Again, delivery is to be effected by anointing. Presumably the midwife manually dilates the womb to allow the head to come through. In the fourth example, one has to rely on the illustration because the text is not clear. The writer simply says that if the child presents unnaturally the mother is to be put in a short, straight, hard bed of "hygh stondyng." That this bed is the birth chair which dated from antiquity and continued in use until the seventeenth century seems unlikely. Soranus describes the birth-stool as follows:

> For normal labor one must prepare beforehand . . . "a midwife's stool," in order that the laboring woman may be placed in position upon it. In the middle of the stool and in the part where they [the midwives] give support one must have cut out a crescent-shaped cavity of medium size, neither too big so that the woman sinks down to the hips, nor, on the contrary, narrow so that the vagina is compressed. The latter is the more troublesome, for the excessively wide hole can be filled up, if she [the midwife] puts pieces of cloth between. And the entire width of the whole stool must be sufficient to accommodate relatively fleshy women too; and its height medium, for in women of small size a footstool placed beneath makes up the deficiency. [II. 2–3]

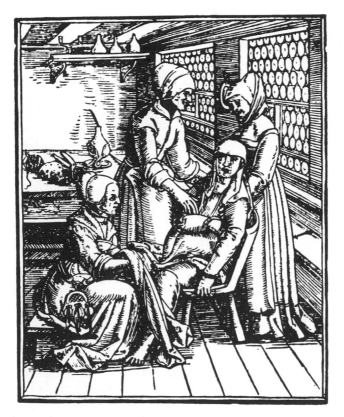

The birth-room in Jacob Rueff's *Ein schön lustig Trostbüchle*, 1554.

Between the fourteenth and fifteenth centuries, the stool of the earlier period appears to have developed into a chair with back and sides. Rösslin provided illustrations of it and stated that it should not be higher than two feet from the ground. The direction in our manuscript that the woman lying on the bed is to "put out her head" suggests the possibility that she is required to lie *crosswise* on the bed. The illustration is of a transverse lie and the writer provides a method of dealing with any irregularity. Celsus seems to have been the first to describe and use what is now known as the Walcher position, in which the woman lies transversely across the bed, her buttocks raised and placed right at the edge so that her legs hang down: "In the first place, 'tis proper to lay the woman on her back across a bed, in such a posture that her ilia may be compressed by her thighs: whence it happens that both the bottom of her belly is presented to the view of the physician and the child is forced to the mouth of the womb."[117]

In the instance described by Celsus, the purpose was to extract a dead fetus. Soranus also recommended a bed when the fetus did not respond to manual traction and had to be extracted by hooks:

> Put the whole patient in a sloping position [upon a bed] which is relatively hard, so that the loins are not allowed to sink in. With the thighs parted and drawn toward the abdomen, she should prop herself with her feet against the bedstead. Then one should have her held fast on either side by servants; but if such are not present, one should fasten down her thorax to the bed by means of a bandage, so that the body of the patient cannot follow the extraction of the fetus. [IV. 9]

It seems likely that our writer is advising the first position rather than the second. In difficult cases, the pelvis is to be tilted in order to facilitate delivery. The fifth and sixth cases also concern the transverse lie. In the fifth example, the transverse lie is to be turned into a head presentation, a procedure that could only be successful if the membranes were not ruptured. In such cases, a Cesarean would now be performed, except in the case of the second of twins. The seventh case is a prolapsed-foot presentation or a transverse presentation, and the recommendation is to bring down both feet but not to pull too soon. A similar recommendation is made in connection with the eighth case, which is a double footling presentation, and with cases nine and ten, which are also footling presentations. In the tenth case, the illustration does not fit the text. The illustration shows the child with arms flexed at the elbow and slightly raised on either side. In the text, the problem is said to be "if the child show first forth his feet apart and his one hand between his feet and his head hanging backwards." The eleventh case is a shoulder presentation, and the advice "to bring down as a head presentation" is reasonable. Today, the child would probably be delivered as a footling or by Cesarean. The twelfth case is "if a child show first forth his knees bent." The situation described is that of a footling breech. The legs are flexed, and the midwife is urged to try and alter the situation by correcting the feet and general posture. Such recommendations would not be practical, and even the adviser appears to think that the grace of God as well as the midwife's skill is required for a successful delivery in this instance.

In the remaining cases, the birth figures do not precisely illustrate the text. In some instances, the reason for the incongruity may not be far to seek. When an inverted flask represents the womb, as in most of the Muscio manuscripts, the mouth of it clearly represents the mouth of the uterus; when a circle is used, as in this manuscript, the mouth of the womb is not indicated, and an illustration can easily be incorrectly placed. In the thirteenth case, a transverse lie is depicted in the illustration, but the description appears to concern a frank breech. The midwife is instructed to bring the foot down and break up the breech. The fourteenth case also appears to describe a frank breech, but the illustration is of a head presentation with prolapsed foot and hand. Here one might indeed question whether the illustration has been properly placed. If the opening of the vagina were on the right, the illustration would be correct, showing a frank breech. The fifteenth case appears to involve a major complication—"if the child lies prostrate or else upright and his feet and his hands are over his head." Here the illustration (which is out of position) presents a frank breech. Delivery by the head is recommended. The sixteenth case deals with multiple births—"if there were more than one as it happens every day and all of them come to the orifice at once." This case is accompanied by two illustrations, the first showing twins with footling presentation and the second showing twins with headling presentation. Such a situation can only happen with premature twins, otherwise two heads do not appear together. A situation can arise when one twin comes by the buttocks and one by the head, and as a result the two heads get locked;[118] perhaps this situation is being referred to here.

The instructions are remarkable for their detail, and they appear to be the starting place in the vernacular for recommendations that are to be repeated not only in *The Byrth of Mankynde* but in more popular chapbooks, such as *Aristotle's Masterpiece*, with its sensational old wives' tales and cautionary woodcuts. The edition of *Aristotle's Masterpiece* for 1690, for example, which was regarded as "very necessary for all Midwives, Muses and Young Married Women," describes many of the fetal positions given in Sloane 2463 and offers similar advice on how to adjust the child in the womb.

The question arises: how was this manuscript preserved? It is one of a collection of four medical tracts that once belonged to Richard Ferris, Master of the Barbers' and Surgeons' Company in 1563 and Sergeant Surgeon to Queen Elizabeth. At his death it passed to John Feld, who paid the executors forty-eight shillings and fourpence for it. In the collection are a work on anatomy also decorated and in the hand of a professional scribe (ff. 1–51v); a second work of ninety-five chapters dealing with the composition of the blood, treatment of wounds, apostemes, eye troubles, broken bones, and internal ruptures (ff. 53–152); a third text of seven chapters, introduced as "the book the whiche is clepid the antitodarie," an assortment of recipes and treatments on the same topics, including diseases of the eye (ff. 154–93v), with a definite conclusion: "Now is the time to make an end," and a left margin notation: "perfecto libro, February 27, 1585," and the present gynecological treatise. Presumably all four were once separate entities.

Sloane 2463 is on vellum, the folios being 7 1/2 inches in breadth and 10 1/2 inches in depth. It is written in the hand of a professional scribe of the early fifteenth century, with 32 lines to a page. On the first folio, figure 202 has been crossed out and replaced by 194. The next folios are numbered 2–6 and these have been crossed out and replaced by numbers 195–199. After folio 6, there is only the later numbering, ending at folio 232. Presumably the well-defined chapter headings originally made the pagination unnecessary. The treatise ends abruptly, and folio 233v contains two recipes for jaundice in a sixteenth-century hand. In all four manuscripts, several later hands have made brief marginal headings. Different seventeenth-century hands have made headings in thin ink in the gynecological manuscript. The handwriting, for example, of "menstrua stopped" at the top of ff. 196v, 197, and "menstruis stopped" at the top of 19v, 198, appears to differ from that of "menstruis stopped" at the top of ff. 198v, 199. There are also some short headings in red in a fifteenth-century hand.

This manuscript is more splendidly decorated than the others. The first folio, which is well worn, has the initial F decorated, 2 inches by 2 inches in its widest part with elaborate fronds of foliation in brown, blue, pink, and green stretching vertically and horizontally to the margins of the page. The initial itself is blue embossed with gold, and pink and green colors are used in the background foliation. On the same page, red is used to delineate a new paragraph. The scribe used the same sign to denote paragraphing throughout the work, coloring it either blue or red. In the enumeration of the chapters, on folio 195, and sometimes as an indication of the end of a chapter in the text, a decoration is used thus:

with the top line in red and the bottom in blue or the reverse. Initials to chapters are blue with a background of red penwork with featherlike decoration extending into the left margin. In some instances the chapter headings are in larger letters, or they are in red or are underlined in red.

As I have already indicated, other manuscripts contain passages similar to those in Sloane 2463. Sloane 5, handsomely written on vellum with red initials, has the familiar opening on f. 158, "Sires we shull understonde . . . ," and deals with "Grevaunce that women have in berynge of childrene" (f. 165), concluding on f. 172v with "bledynge of the moder." It then goes on to astrology, and omits the birth figures that are such a remarkable feature of Sloane 2463. Similarly, BL Royal 18 A. VI, ff. 35–54, is a briefer version of the Sloane manuscript, with chapters in a different order and with no illustrations. It does not give the various fetal positions in detail and concludes, as in the case of Sloane 5, with recipes for women who have lost blood. Unadorned, in a scribal hand, the work contains some crude attempts to color initials in dark red. A slightly more handsome manuscript beginning "Her folowyth the knowyng of womans kynde," with rubrics in red is to be found in BL Additional MS, 12195, ff. 157–85.

Two manuscripts that closely resemble Sloane 2463 are Sloane 249 and MS 129a.i.5 at the Royal College of Surgeons. Sloane 249 has no elegance and is without decoration. Some of the headings to the chapters are in larger lettering, sometimes irregular and with more abbreviations than are used by our scribe. There are alterations and insertions, mainly by later hands. The content of the treatise in Sloane 249, beginning at f. 180v, closely resembles that in our manuscript, and ends abruptly on f. 205v, where it provides a further recipe for the stone and subsequently ascribes the material to Trotula. Whereas Sloane 249 is on parchment, the manuscript at the Royal College of Surgeons is on vellum, approximately six inches wide and eight-and-a-half inches deep, and is written in an elegant scribal hand. Badly stained, it is headed by a distinctive red rubric "Hic incipit liber Trotularis" in different lettering, possibly of the same period. Initials of capitals are decorated with strokes of the same red. On f. 43, "Ad mulieres tantum" forms a rubric in red. In Sloane 2463, f. 228v, the same words have been enlarged and a red line drawn underneath them. On f. 45v, at the bottom, there is a large rubric in red, "Wytnys Trotula," words that appear on f. 230v of Sloane 2463. References that seem local and specify persons and places are the same in all three manuscripts. Certain errors of spelling are repeated: for example, "isapis" for "iaspis," or jasper; "gosti gotes" instead of "gos other"; "anathasia" for "athanasia." [119]

On the other hand, the manuscripts also show discrepancies that arose in the copying. On f. 202, Sloane 2463, the scribe has crossed out a repetition that is allowed to stand in Sloane 249, ff. 186–186v, and in MS 129a.i.5, f. 10v. Two recipes following consecutively are identical save for the opening phrase, the first being "Take lynesede al hole and sethe," the second being "Take lynesede al and sethe." Evidently the scribe of Sloane 2463 realized that the second recipe was unnecessary after he had copied it. It is expunged by a thin red line with dots underneath in a paler ink. The two other manuscripts have not expunged the duplicated recipe, and MS 129a.i.5 includes "hole" in the repetition. These manuscripts are clearly copies made by scribes not competent in the medical field. The original treatise, bringing together empiric remedies of the time and translations or adaptations from the accepted corpus of medieval medical texts, must have been compiled by someone familiar with the earlier authorities and proficient in the medical art. Later, in the hands of scribes, some parts of the compilation were misunderstood and copied imperfectly, especially those portions that had been left in Latin.

That these copies were based on an English text is suggested by the various local allusions to which we have already referred. The copy at the Royal College of Surgeons, with its title "Hic Incipit Liber Trotularis," gives the text further identification. Sloane 2463, together with the other copies of an undiscovered earlier text, is the English Trotula. Thoroughly domesticated and different from the Latin Trotula, it nevertheless takes its name from the legendary physician popularly associated with gynecology. Through this work, instructions for treating women's ailments, combining recipes and practices from ancient literary sources with those derived from oral tradition, were widely disseminated, and as the basis for the earliest gynecological printed text, they dictated childbirth procedures for many centuries.

# NOTES

1. *De Recuperatione Terre Sancte*, ed. Ch.-V. Langlois, pp. 51–52, 70–71. Pierre Dubois was, however, no feminist: the medical course was to be simplified because of the "inferiority" of women.

2. Tacitus, *The Annals*, XII, lxvi–vii.

3. *Hygini Fabulae*, ed. M. Schmidt, p. 150 [CCLXXIV]: " . . . quae cum credere se noluisset existimans virum esse illa tunica sublata ostendebat se foeminam esse." Because it occurs among references to Cheiron, Apollo, and Daedalus, however, the story may be apocryphal.

4. Martial, *Epigrams*, XI, lxxi; Josephus, *Life*, I, 18.

5. A. Hübner, *Inscriptiones Hispaniae Latinae*, p. 62, no. 497.

6. Tacitus, *De Origine et Situ Germanorum*, VII, 4.

7. *Gynaecea ad Saluinam*, p. 136: "Saluina, artis meae dulce ministerium. . . .

8. *Aetios of Amida*, trans. James V. Ricci, p. 12; XVIII, LI, XCVII, C, CII, CVI.

9. Venantius Fortunatus, "Vita Sanctae Radegundis," p. 39.

10. George L. Hamilton, *MP*, 4 (1906), 3. The popularity of Trotula's work is also suggested by its appearance in translation in the first part of an Irish gynecological text in a scrapbook of Irish medical tracts made, according to the compiler, in 1352. See *Irish Texts, Fasciculus V*, ed. J. Fraser et al.

11. *The Diseases of Women by Trotula of Salerno*, trans. Elizabeth Mason-Hohl, p. x.

12. Cols. 215–16.

13. *Trotula*, p. x. Elizabeth Mason-Hohl does not cite a source for her contention. On Trotula, see also Mélanie Lipinska, *Histoire des Femmes Médicins depuis l'Antiquité jusqu'à nos Jours*, pp. 86–89; Kate Campbell Hurd-Mead, *A History of Women in Medicine*, pp. 136–37; "Trotula," *Isis*, 14 (1930), 349; H. P. Bayon, *Proc. RSM*, 33 (1939–40), 471–75; H. P. Cholmeley, *John of Gaddesden and the "Rosa Medicinae,"* appendix E, p. 183; Charles and Dorothea Singer, "The Origin of the Medical School of Salerno, the First University. An Attempted Reconstruction," *Essays on the History of Medicine Presented to Karl Sudhoff*, p. 129; Muriel Joy Hughes, *Women Healers in Medieval Life and Literature*, pp. 101–6; *Irish Texts, Fasciculus V*, ed. J. Fraser et al., pp. xv–xix.

14. The observations given here on the origins of Trotula are condensed from three public lectures that I gave on "Trotula of Salerno and the works attributed to her" at the Adam Mickiewicz University, Poland, October 4, 1975, University of British Columbia, November 14, 1975, and the University of Southern Tennessee, April 16, 1977. Edward F. Tuttle, "The *Trotula* and Old Dame Trot: A Note on the Lady of Salerno," *Bull. Hist. of Med.*, 50 (1976), 61–72, deals with the same material and reaches conclusions very similar to my own. I therefore refer the reader to this excellent article. On this subject, see also T. J. Garbáty, "Chaucer's Weaving Wife," *JAF*, 81 (1968), 342–46; William Matthews, "The Wife of Bath and All Her Sect," *Viator*, 5 (1974), 413–43; B. Rowland, "Exhuming Trotula, *Sapiens Matrona* of Salerno," *Florilegium*, 1 (1979), 42–57.

15. *Pamphile et Galatée*, ed. Joseph de Morawski, p. 137. For subsequent use, see *OED*, sv. *Trot*. v. 2.

16. Godefroy, VIII, 92.

17. Albertus Magnus, "Metaphysica," IV, i, 6, *Opera Omnia*, XVI, i, 169: "illa vero alia dicuntur nomine illo faciendo actionem aliquam illius, sicut vetula dicitur medica"; St. Bernardino, "Selecta ex autographo Budapestinen-si," *Opera Omnia*, IX, 369: "O medici, studuistis in gramatica, logica, philosophia, medicina, cum multis spensis, periculis et laboribus; a la vechi [a] rinchagnata n'à l'onore!" The subject of one of Trotula's recipes is found in Galen, *Opera*, ed. C. G. Kuhn, XIV, 478: *Ut mulier violata appareat virgo*.

18. P. 75.

19. P. 40. See also J. O. Halliwell, *A Dictionary of Archaic and Provincial Words*, II, sv. *Trot*.

20. George Sarton, *Introduction to the History of Science*, I, 283.

21. For Salerno, see P. O. Kristeller, *Bull. Hist. Med.*, 17 (1945), 148.

22. Percy Flemming, *Proc. RSM*, 22 (1928–29), 771–82; *Customary of Benedictine Monasteries of St. Augustine, Canterbury, and St. Peter, Westminster*, ed. E. Maunde Thompson, pp. 297, 300, 325–32; see also Loren C. MacKinney, *Medical Illustrations in Medieval Manuscripts*, pp. 3–4; James V. Ricci, *The Genealogy of Gynaecology*, p. 207. For study of clerical involvement in medical practice, see D. W. Amundsen, "Medieval Canon Law . . . ," *Bull. Hist. Med.*, 52 (1978), 22–44.

23. M. R. James, *The Ancient Libraries of Canterbury and Dover*, p. 481, no. 347; p. 482, no. 355. Christchurch Library has *Practica domine Trote ad prouocanda menstrua* (p. 58, no. 475) and under *Practica Johannis de Platea* includes *Tractatus de ornatu mulierum, liber de egritudinis* and *liber de curiacionibus mulierum* (p. 59). The catalogue of the library of St. Augustine's shows *Cleopatra de ornatu mulierum* and refers to various works on women's diseases (p. 335), *Trotula* (p. 339, no. 1219, 6), (p. 340, no. 1225, 7), and *trotule* (p. 345, no. 1255). In the collection of John of London is *trotula maior et minor* (p. 385, no. 1599). See also pp. 480–84 for books of Dover Priory listing *Trotula maior de pas'* (p. 481, no. 347), *Trotula Maior* (p. 482, no. 355).

24. Rotha Mary Clay, *The Mediaeval Hospitals of England*, pp. 25, 82, 83.

25. Ed. Paul Kaiser, Leipzig, 1903. See also G. M. Engbring, "Saint Hildegard, Twelfth-Century Physician," *Bull. Hist. Med.*, 8 (1940), 770–84.

26. "Vita Sanctae Hildegardis auctoribus Godefrido et Theodorico," *PL*, 197, cols. 91 ff., esp. cols. 118, 119.

27. *Pierce the Ploughmans Crede*, ed. W. W. Skeat, l.703.

28. See George Stephens, *Archaeologia*, 30 (1844), 417; Rossell Hope Robbins, *Speculum*, 45 (1970), 401.

29. *Tristan und Isolt* by Gottfried von Strassburg, ed. August Cross, l.1276.

30. Ed. E. Kölbing, ll. 3671–73. On women physicians in fiction, see Ida B. Jones, *Bull. Inst. Hist. Med.*, 5 (1937), 421; M. J. Hughes, *Women Healers*, pp. 30, 33, 98.

31. P. 184. On medieval women and the practice of medicine, see also Eileen Power, "The Position of Women," in *The Legacy of the Middle Ages*, 1926, ed. Charles George Crump and E. F. Jacob, p. 421.

32. Joshua Trachtenburg, *Jewish Magic and Superstition*, pp. 4–7.

33. G. L. Kriegk, *Deutsches Bürgerthum im Mittelalter*, I, passim.

34. *Chartularum universitatis Parisiensis*, ed. P. Heinrich Denifle, II, 149–50

(Clarice de Rothomago); II, 255–67 (Jacqueline Felicie de Almania). For plea, see II, 264: "Item melius est et honestius et par quod mulier sagax et experta in arte visitet mulierem infirmam, videatque et inquirat secreta nature et abscondita ejus, quam homo, cui non licet predicta videre, inquirere, nec palpare manus, mammas, ventrem et pedes, etc., mulierum; imo debet homo mulierum secreta et earum societas secretas evitare et fugere quantum potest. Et mulier antea permitteret se mori, quam secreta infirmitatis sue homini revelare propter honestatem et propter verecundiam, quam revelando pateretur." See also Ernest Wickersheimer, *Commentaires de la Faculté de Médicine de l'université de Paris* (1395–1516), I, 317. See also his commentary, pp. lxxii–v. For the dating of various university faculties in Europe, see P. Heinrich Denifle, *Die Entstehung der Universitäten des Mittelalters bis 1400*, I, 807–10. See also Pearl Kibre, *Bull. Hist. Med.*, 27 (1953), 7–12; M. J. Hughes, *Women Healers*, pp. 89–92.

35. See C. H. Talbot and E. A. Hammond, *The Medical Practitioners in Mediaeval England*, passim.

36. *Rotuli Parliamentorum* (London, 1783), IV, 158.

37. *Promptorium Parvulorum*, p. 163.

38. *Speculum*, 45 (1970), 394.

39. Camb. Univ. MS I. 6, 33, f. 33.

40. *The English Register of Godstow Nunnery, near Oxford*, ed. A. Clark, pt. i, p. 25; *The Myroure of oure Ladye*, ed. John Henry Blunt, pp. xl, 2.

41. *Speculum*, 45 (1970), 413.

42. *Causae et Curae*, ed. P. Kaiser, pp. 17–18, 77–78, 97. Soranus stated that the moon had no influence (I.x.41). For physicians' tables, see C. H. Talbot, "A Mediaeval Physician's Vade Mecum," *J. Hist. Med. & Al. Scs.*, 16 (1961), 213–33; Loren C. MacKinney, *Medical Illustrations*, p. 21; Rossell Hope Robbins, "Mirth in Manuscripts," *E&S*, 21 (1968), 8. For the subsequent disappearance of astrology from orthodox medicine in the seventeenth century, see Keith Thomas, *Religion and the Decline of Magic*, p. 354.

43. Trans. Henry E. Sigerist. *Quart. Bull. Northwestern Univ. Medic. School*, 20 (1946), 136–43.

44. See C. F. Meyer, *Bull. Hist. Med.*, 7 (1939), 389.

45. *The Cyrurgie of Guy de Chauliac*, ed. Margaret Ogden, p. 10.

46. *Treatises of Fistula in Ano*, ed. D'Arcy Power, p. 44.

47. *Opera Omnia*, III, proem.

48. P. Horton-Smith Hartley and H. R. Aldridge, *Johannes de Mirfeld of St. Bartholomew's, Smithfield. His Life and Works*, p. 123. Recipe for gunpowder is on p. 91.

49. Bodleian MS Douce 37, f. 1v.

50. Bm. Royal MS 18 A. VI, f. 55v.

51. Bodley MS 178, f. 151.

52. *Histoire de la Médicine*, I, 431–32. On this subject in Hippocratic times, see Danielle Gourevitch, *Presse Médicale*, 76 (1968), 544–46.

53. P. iv. The works of Nicholas Culpepper (1616–54) have been reprinted many times, his *English Physician and Complete Herbal* as recently as 1961.

54. *The Female Physician*, preface.

55. *A Treatise of the Acute Diseases of Infants . . . written originally in Latin by the late learned Walter Harris M.D.*, p. 76. Harris' own patients experienced

# 52

miraculous recoveries, with the exception of Queen Mary who disregarded his advice and expired after taking Venice treacle recommended by another physician as a cure for smallpox.

56. *The Byrth of Mankynde*, ff. v,vii; see J. W. Ballantyne, *J. Obstet. & Gynaec.*, 10 (1906), 297–325; Palmer Findley, *Med. Life*, 42 (1935), 171–74.

57. W. Smellie, *A Treatise on the Theory and Practice of Midwifery*, pp. xxxv–vi; Aveling, *History*, p. xvi. Aveling published an extract from Sloane 2463, and maintained that "it was proper to commence each subject with its history," *Trans. Obstet. Soc.*, 7 (1867), 374.

58. M. R. James, *Ancient Libraries*, p. 60, no. 496: "liber Soracii [Sorani], phisici ad Cleopatram Reginam de mulieribus."

59. Also extant are parts of translation by Caelius Aurelianus. See *Gynaecia*, eds. M. F. and I. E. Drabkin; Brian Lawn, *The Salernitan Question*, p. 5n.

60. Trans. James V. Ricci, pp. 30–31. Cf. Albucasis, *Fragmenta*, ff. 193–99.

61. J. T. Noonan, Jr., *Contraception*, p. 213, notes that "there is nothing to indicate that an ordinary physician would not have considered contraception a sin."

62. *Breuiarium Practice*, III, iv: "Sed contra naturam & pedibus retortis, vel stans reversus & sic inde reducatur ad unum de duobus modis ab obstetrice, ut sit cum capite vel pedibus ante & cum brachiis plicatis ut decet exeat naturaliter exitu." Arnaldus attributes some of his advice to "vetula Salerni."

63. XVI, xxxiii.

64. *Speculum Doctrinale*, XIV, cxxvi, cols., 1364–65.

65. *Cyrurgie*, p. 530 [my translation].

66. *Practica*, fols. 220v ff.; *Compendium Medicine*, fols. 290ff.; *Breuiarium Practice*, III; *Fragmenta* in *Gynaecorum*, cols. 193–99.

67. "Surcester" for "Cirencester" was in use 1412–39. See *Place Names of Gloucestershire*, I, 60.

68. See entries in *The Oath Book or Red Parchment Book of Colchester*, trans. W. Gurney Benham, pp. 7, 9.

69. *Middle English Dictionary*, sv. *March* n. 2 (5); *light-fot* adj. The names are not recorded in C. H. Talbot and E. A Hammond, *The Medical Practitioners in Mediaeval England*.

70. Bernard Ward, *St. Edmund*, p. 169 [Cambridge MS].

71. Ibid., p. 181 [Faustine MS]; see also A. T. Baker, *Rom.*, 55 (1929), 379, ll. 1940–64 [Welbeck MS]; C. H. Lawrence, *St. Edmund of Abingdon*, pp. 101–5.

72. Handwritten MS at the Academy of Medicine, Toronto.

73. *Culpepper's Compleat and Experienc'd Midwife in Two Parts*, p. 36.

74. *Generation of Animals*, trans. A. L. Peck, I, xix–xx.

75. "De Genesi ad Litteram," *PL*, 34, cols. 421–22.

76. *De Coitu*, trans. Paul Delany, *ChauR*, 4 (1970), 56. Cf. St. Hildegard, *Causae et Curae*, pp. 104, 109.

77. I, x, 36. See also exposition by J. H. Waszink in his edition of Tertullian's *De Anima*, pp. 342–46; for a recent discussion see Vern L. Bullough, *Viator*, 4 (1973), 485–501; Henry Hargreaves, "De spermate hominis," *MS*, 39 (1977), 506–10.

78. G. Henslow, *Medical Works of the Fourteenth Century*, p. 32.

79. *Ein mittelenglisches Medizinbuch*, ed. F. Heinrich, pp. 143–44. See also Douglas Gray, "Notes on Some Middle English Charms," in *Chaucer and Middle English Studies in Honour of Rossell Hope Robbins*, pp. 56–71.

53

80. James Raine, *Fabric Rolls of York Minster*, p. 260: "exercet officium obstetricis . . . utitur etiam incantationibus."

81. W. H. Frère, ed. *Visitations*, II, 59ff.

82. *The Remains of Edmund Grindal*, ed. W. Nicholson, p. 174.

83. Myrc, *Instructions for Parish Priests*, ll. 97–101.

84. Frère, ed. *Visitations*, II, 58, n.2.

85. Adolphe de Chesnel, *Dictionnaire des Superstitions, erreurs, préjugés, et traditions populaires*, cols. 733–34; T. R. Forbes, *The Midwife and the Witch*, pp. 96 ff.

86. *Customary of the Benedictine Monasteries of St. Augustine, Canterbury and St. Peter, Westminster*, ed. E. Maunde Thompson, II, 73.

87. Ed. W. W. Skeat, p. 4, ll. 78–79.

88. Frère, *Visitations*, II, 58, n. 2.

89. *Letters on Demonology and Witchcraft*, p. 126.

90. Curt F. Bühler, *Speculum*, 39 (1964), 274.

91. Adolphe de Chesnel, *Dictionnaire*, col. 896.

92. M. Höfler, *Volksmedizin und Aberglaube*, p. 39.

93. Forbes, p. 68.

94. *Culpepper*, 3rd ed., pp. 55–56.

95. Campbell Bonner, *Studies in Magical Amulets, Chiefly Graeco-Egyptian*, pp. 79–83; E. A. Budge, *Amulets and Superstitions*, pp. 314–30.

96. *English Mediaeval Lapidaries*, ed. J. Evans and M. S. Sergeantson, p. 121; Albertus Magnus, *Book of Minerals*, trans. Dorothy Wykoff, p. 100.

97. *PL*, 197, col. 1257.

98. Höfler, *Volksmedizin*, p. 39.

99. Ed. Kühn, XIV, 476.

100. *Culpepper*, p. 133.

101. *NH*, XXVIII, 248–49; J. Delcourt, *Medicina de Quadrupedibus*, pp. 12, 22–27.

102. Abortion as a moral issue is still subject to divergent opinions in the Church. See *Theol. Stud.*, 31 (1970), 3–176.

103. Francesco Roberti, comp., *Dictionary of Moral Theology*, p. 6.

104. For detailed information on patristic, scholastic, and papal statements on abortion, see J. T. Noonan, Jr., *Nat. Law Forum*, 12 (1967), 88–131; Herbert Waddams, *Dictionary of Christian Ethics*, sv. "Abortion." Augustine's theory is well explained by George H. Williams, *Theol. Stud.*, 31 (1970), 26–28.

105. Joseph F. Donceel, *Theol. Stud.*, 31 (1970), 78–85.

106. *De Anima*, XXV, iv: "Atquin et in ipso adhuc utero infans trucidatur, necessaria crudelitate, cum in exitu obliquatus denegat partum, matricida ni moriturus."

107. *De Eccl. Disciplinis*, II, lxxxix, *PL*, 132, col. 301: "Si aliquis causa explendae libidinis, vel odii meditatione, ut non ex eo soboles nascatur, homini aut mulieri aliquid fecerit, vel ad potandum dederit ut non possit generare aut concipere, ut homicida teneatur."

108. II, Bk.I. cap. xxiii, "De Homicidio."

109. " . . . occisio puerorum ante baptismum eorum procuracio aborcii aut destruccio seminum ante formatum fetum facta per medicinas sint grauia peccata ualde." H. S. Cronin, *EHR*, 22 (1907), 303. See also Chaucer, *ParsT*, 575 ff.

110. Brussels, Bibliothèque Royale, MS 3714, ff. 26v–29 [Codex Bruxellensis]; Copenhagen, Kongelige Bibliotek, MS G.K.S. 1653, 4⁰, ff. 17–19

[Codex Hafniensis]; MS Thott, 190. 2º, f. 6; Dresden, Sächsische Landesbibliothek MS P. 34, ff. 212–15v; Erlangen, Universitätsbibliothek, MS B 200, ff. 78–79; MS B 33, 93v–95; Leipzig, Universitätsbibliothek, MS 1192, ff. 263v–64v; London, British Library, MS Sloane 249, ff. 196v–97v; Royal College of Surgeons, MS 129a.i.5, ff. 28v–31; Montpellier, Bibliothèque de l'école de Médicin, MS 277, ff. 162–63v; Oxford, Bodleian Library, MS Ashmole 399, ff. 14–15; MS Laud 724, ff. 97–97v; Paris, Bibliothèque Nationale, MS Lat. 7056, ff. 87–89; Rome, Bibliotheca Apostolica Vaticana, MS Pal. Lat. 1304, ff. 83–84v; Stockholm, Kungliga Biblioteket, MS X. 118; Venice, Biblioteca Nazionale Marciana, MS Lat. Z. 320 (1937), f. 98; Munich, Bayerische Staatsbibliothek, MS 597, ff. 259v–61v.

111. See E. Ingerslev, *J. Obstet. & Gynaec.*, 15 (1909), 25.

112. Stockholm, Kungliga Biblioteket, MS X.118 (1412), in center column, positions 10–20.

113. However, a Middle English rhyming poem in a fifteenth–century hand compares the embryo to a hare sitting on its form, and describes the fetal position more realistically, using the word *bowyd*: bent, curved. See Hargreaves, "De spermate hominis," *MS*, 39 (1977), 507.

114. Bodleian MS Laud 724, f. 97.

115. *Speculum Doctrinale*, XIV, cxxvi, cols. 1364–65.

116. I should like to express my thanks to Dr. Gwyn Stuart Thomas of Calgary for his observations on the birth figures.

117. Trans. James Grieve, p. 455. *De Medicina*, vii, 29: "Oportet autem ante omnia resupinam mulierem transverso lecto sic collocare, ut feminibus eius ipsius ilia comprimatur; quo fit, ut et imus venter in conspectu medici sit et infans ad os volvae conpellatur."

118. *Obstetrics*, ed. J. P. Greenhill, p. 630; R. Szwarcberg, P. H. Houyet, and B. Keller, "Accrochage de jumeaux: une circonstance obstétricale exceptionnelle," *Rev. franç. Gynéc.*, 68 (1973), 59–62; G. Kuppe, "Zwillingskollision mit Kinn-zu-Kinn-Verhakung," *Zentralblatt fuer Gynaekologie*, 95 (1973), 583–86.

119. Sloane 2463, ff. 221, 211v, 203v; Sloane 249, ff. 192v, 199, 187v; MS 129a.i.5, ff. 22, 33, 13.

# AN ENGLISH TROTULA MANUSCRIPT, SLOANE 2463, With a Modern English Translation

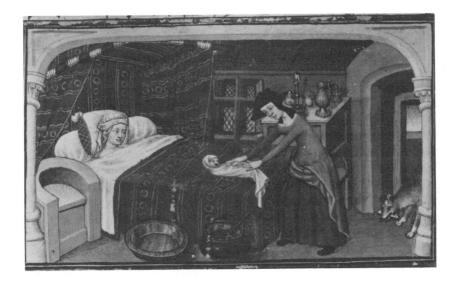

A birth-room scene (MS. Roy 20, B XX, f. 86v).

# NOTE ON THE TEXT

The spelling of Sloane 2463 has been reproduced with as few emendations as possible. The ampersand sign has been retained. Any word added has been placed in square brackets. Abbreviations, contractions, and suspensions have been expanded without italics. In medical prescriptions, three apothecary's symbols have been retained in the text. They are ℥ (ounce), ℨ (drachm), ℈ (scruple). The abbreviation designating half (a long *s* with a backstroke through it, standing for the Latin *semis*) is printed *sem*. Other abbreviations are *li.* (pound) and *m.* (handful).

Illuminated capitals have been indented and are printed in boldface in the text; rubrics and other words or phrases that were underlined or written large in either text or margins are italicized. Marginal notations in sixteenth- and seventeenth-century hands have not been transcribed, because they appear only in the initial section of the manuscript. Paragraph signs have been shown by moving directly to the left margin of the next line in the text; paragraph indentations have been added at appropriate places in the facing translation for readability. The chapter-listing on folio 195r is obviously indented in the manuscript and has been copied exactly. Latin case endings have been, in general, preserved exactly as they appear in the manuscript, even though this sometimes results in a mixing of genitives and accusatives in recipes, and in unusual constructions for other sentence parts. In translating the manuscript from early fifteenth-century to modern English, the aim has been to produce a readable text, retaining something of its quaintness and charm, while keeping the sense of the original.

58

[f. 194r] For as moche as ther ben manye women that hauen many diuers maladies and sekenesses nygh* to þe deth and thei also ben shamefull to schewen and to tellen her greuaunces unto eny wyght, therfor I schal sumdele wright to herre maladies remedye, praying to God ful of grace to sende me grace truly to write to þe plesaunce of God & to all womannes helpyng. For charite axeth this: that euery man schuld trauaille for helpyng of his brotheryn & his susteryn after þe grace of God þat he hathe vnderfongyn. And thowgh women have diuers evelles & many greet greuaunces mo than all men knowen of, as I seyd, hem schamen for drede of repreving in tymes comyng & of discuryng off vncurteys men þat loue women but for her lustes and for her foule lykyng. And yf women be in dissese, suche men haue hem in despyte & thenke nought how moche dysese women haue or þan they haue brought hem into þis world. And therfore, in helping of women I wyl wright of women prevy sekenes the helpyng, and that oon woman may helpe another in her syke-nesse & nought diskuren her previtees to suche vncurteys men. But neuertheles, whosoeuer he be þat displesith a woman for herr sekenesse þat sche hath of þe ordynaunce of God, he doth a gret synne. For he dispisith nought allonely hem but God that sendith hem suche sekenesse for her best. And þerfore no man shuld dispise oþer for þe disese þat God sendith hym but to haue compassion of hym and releuen hym yef he myght.

[f. 194v] Therfore ye schal vnderstonde that women haue lesse hete in here bodies þan men haue and more moistnesse for defaute of hete þat shuld dryen her moistnesse & her humors, but netheles of bledyng to make her bodies clene & hoole from syknesse. And they haue such purgacions from tyme of twelue wynter age into þe age of fyfty wynter. But nethelesse somme women haue it longer as þei þat ben of high complexion & beth norisshed with hote metes & wit hote drynkes & leven in moche reste. And they haue this purgacion in euery moneth ones but it be women þat be with childe or ellis women þat be of drie complexion & trauayle moche. For women after þei be with child for to they be deliuered, thei ne haue nought þis purgacion for þe

*nygh: MS. nyhg.

[f. 194r]  Because there are many women who have numerous diverse illnesses—some of them almost fatal—and because they are also ashamed to reveal and tell their distress to any man, I therefore shall write somewhat to cure their illnesses, praying to merciful God to send me grace to write truly to His satisfaction and to the assistance of all women. For charity calls for this: that everyone should work to help his brothers and sisters according to the grace that he has received of God. And although women have various maladies and more terrible sicknesses than any man knows, as I said, they are ashamed for fear of reproof in times to come and of exposure by discourteous men who love women only for physical pleasure and for evil gratification. And if women are sick, such men despise them and fail to realize how much sickness women have before they bring them into this world. And so, to assist women, I intend to write of how to help their secret maladies so that one woman may aid another in her illness and not divulge her secrets to such discourteous men.

But nevertheless, whoever he be that offends a woman because of the malady that she has by God's command, commits a great sin; for he despises not only women but God who sends such sickness in their best interests. And therefore no one should despise another for the disease that God sends but should have compassion and help if he can.

[f. 194v]  Therefore, you must understand that women have less heat in their bodies than men and have more moisture because of lack of heat that would dry their moisture and their humors, but nevertheless they have bleeding which makes their bodies clean and whole from sickness. And they have such purgations from the age of twelve to fifty. Even so, some women have purgations for a longer time because they are of a high complexion and are nourished with hot food and drink and live in much ease. And they have this purgation once every month unless they are pregnant or are of a dry complexion and work hard. For women, from the time that they are with child until they are delivered, do not have this purgation, because the childe in her wombe is norisshed with þe blood þat þei shuld be purged of. And yf thei haue purgacion in this tyme it is a token þat þe child refusith þat blood and than that childe is fallen into sume sikenesse or it wyl dey in his moder wombe. Women þat be of an high complexion & faren wel & leven in moche ease hauen this purgacion ofter þan ones in a moneth. And this blode þat passith from women in tyme of hir purgacion cometh ouȝte of þe veynes þat ben in þe marice that is cleped the moder & norisscher to þe childern riȝt conceyved in hem. The moder is a skyn þat þe childe is enclosed in his moder wombe. And many off þe seke- nesses that women hauen comen of grevaunces of this moder that we clepen the marice.

The first is stoppyng of the blode that thei [f. 195r] sculde haue in her purgacion & be purged, as I haue sayde.

The seconde is to moche flowyng of suche blode & in vntyme. And that syknesse febleth women full moche.

The thirde sykenesse is suffocacion of þe moder.

The fyrth is precipitacion of þe moder.

The fyfte is whan þe moder is flawe fro withinforth.

The sixte is whan þer is a posteme of þe moder.

The seuenth is þe swellyng of þe moder.

The eght is of trauaylyng that women haue in þe childyng, and the harde greuaunces that they haue or they ben delyuered.

The nynthe is the goyng oute of the moder benethenforthe.

The tenth is withholdyng of the secundine and ache of the moder.

*The fyrst chapiter is of þe stoppyng of her blode þat they shuld haue in her purgacions & be purged off.*

Withholdyng of this blode that þei mowe noȝt haue her purga- cions in due tymes comyn in diuerse maners and of diuerse enchesons: as of hete ether of colde of þe moder; other of hete oþer of colde of þe humours þat be enclosed withynforth in þe moder; other of gret drynesse of her complexion, other of moche wakyng, oþer of moche thenkyng, oþer of gret angre, oþer of moche sorowe, oþer of moche fastyng. Signes & tokenes gen-

child in the womb is nourished with the blood instead. And if
they have a purgation at this time, it is a sign that the child
refuses the blood and is sick or will die in its mother's womb.
Women who are of a high complexion and are prosperous and
live in comfort have this purgation more than once a month.
And this blood that passes from women at the time of their
purgation comes out of the veins that are in the uterus that is
called the "mother" and nourishes the children properly
conceived there. The "mother" is a skin in which the child is
enclosed in his mother's womb. And many of the sicknesses that
women have come from the ailments of this "mother"* that we
call the marice [uterus].

The first is concerned with the stopping of the blood that
they [f. 195r] should have in their purgation and be purged of, as
I have said.

The second concerns excessive flowing of such blood and at
the wrong time. And this sickness weakens women very much.

The third sickness is the suffocation of the uterus.

The fourth is the precipitation of the uterus.

The fifth is when the uterus is bruised from within.

The sixth is when there is an inflammation of the uterus.

The seventh is the swelling of the uterus.

The eighth concerns the pain in childbirth and the terrible
suffering women have before they are delivered.

The ninth is the going out of the uterus at the lower part of
the body.

The tenth is the withholding of the secundine and the ache of
the uterus.

*The first chapter is concerned with the stopping of the blood that women should
have in their purgations and be purged of.*

Retention of this blood so that they cannot have their
purgations at the proper time occurs in various ways and for
various reasons: because of the heat or the cold of the uterus or
the heat or cold of the humors that are enclosed inside the
uterus, or excessive dryness of their complexion, or being
awake too much, thinking too much, being too angry or too sad,
or eating too little. Signs and general indications

* Hereafter termed the *uterus*, for purpose of identification. The initial
definition of womb (ll. 25–26) is not maintained throughout the manuscript,
and the word usually serves as a synonym for *marice* and *wombe*.

erall of this syknesse ben these: ache & dolour with greuaunces and hevynesses from þe navel dounward to her prevy membre. And ache of her raynes & of her riggebone & of her foreheved and of þe nekke & of þe eyen & infeccion of þe [f. 195v] bries, that is to say, chaungyng of her colour into another colour than they schuld haue. Also heuynesse aboute þe mouthe of her stomak and ache aboute þe schulder blades bothe before & behynde, & hevynesse of theire thyes & her hyppes & of her hondes & of her legges. And they haue otherwhiles an vnskilfull appetyte to metes þat ben nought accordyng to hem as to eten coles or ryndes or shelles, and her face is evyle ycoloured and oþerwhiles þer wexeth wannesse in her visage. And oþerwhile in þis tyme they haue wille to companye with men & so þei done and bryngen forth chyldren that ben meselles or haue some oþer suche foule syknesse. And longe withholdyng of þis blode makith women otherwhiles to fallen into a dropesye & oþerwhiles makith hem to haue þe emerawdeȝ; otherwhiles it grevith the hert & þe longes and makith hem to haue þe cardiacle. And oþerwhiles it affrayeth þe hert so moche that it makith hem to fallen downe aswowe as though they hadden þe falling evel. And thei liggen in þat syknesse a day or two as though thei wer dede. And oþerwhiles they haue þe scotamie with grete stone-yng in the brayne & wenen þat all thyng tornyth vp so downe. And yf this withholdyng be for the sykenesse of þe blode in þe moder—þat þe blode may not flowe in due tymes, as it schuld—her vryne wyl be otherwhiles rede as blode. And in tyme þat she shuld schewen & in tyme þat she schuld haue her purgacion it wil be dark & the veynes wil be ful of blode & þe colours of her bries, id est, of her chaunginges, than wil be of clere rede.

But yf this withholdyng be of another humour that is hote and drye and is [f. 196r] cleped colre, than they felen brennyng & prykkyng of hete withynforth & her vryne is of an highe coloure & fattye & in tyme of her purgacion a thre dayes or foure that they be delyuered, whan they go to prevy, of a colryk mater that is, as it were, a bronde & her bries ben of swart rede coloure. And yf þis witholdyng be of colde & a moyst humour that is cleped flewme the vryne is fatte & discolored, and in tyme of her purgacion, whan they gone to prevy, they be diliuered of a fleumatike mater that is whiȝt and thykke & her bries ben of feble

of this sickness are these: aching and suffering with physical discomfort and a feeling of weight from the navel down to the privy member. And the ache of their kidneys, backbone, forehead, neck, eyes, and infection of the [f. 195v] waters,* that is to say, their changing into the wrong color. Also heaviness about the mouth of the stomach, aching around the shoulder blades both in front and behind, and heaviness of thighs, hips, hands, and legs. And such women have, at times, an unreasonable appetite for food not suited to them, such as coal or rinds or shells, and their complexion is a bad color or grows pale. And sometimes at this time they have a desire to consort with men and so they do, and produce children that are lepers or have some other such evil sickness. And long retention of this blood occasionally makes women have dropsy or hemorrhoids; or it harms the heart and lungs and produces heart disease. And sometimes it terrifies the heart so much that it causes women to fall down in a faint as though they had the falling sickness. And they lie in that sickness for a day or two as though dead. And sometimes they have dizziness with great confusion in the brain and think that everything is turned upside down. And if this retention is because of sickness of the blood in the uterus—so that the blood does not flow regularly as it should, the woman's urine at times will be as red as blood. And at the time when she should have her purgation the blood will be dark, the veins will be full of blood, and the colors of her waters, that is, of their changing, will then be bright red.

But if this retention is of another humor, that is hot and dry and is [f. 196r] called bile, then women feel burning and pricking of heat inside, and their urine is of a high color and greasy; and at the time of their purgation during the three or four days that they get rid of [the blood], when they go to the privy, they excrete toxic matter like coal, and their waters are dark red. And if this retention is of a cold and moist humor called phlegm, the urine is greasy and discolored, and during purgation, when they go to the privy, they excrete a phlegmatic matter that is white and thick, and their waters are a feeble

* Sherman Kuhn suggested to me that *bries* is the plural of M.E. *bre* (variant *bri*). Sense 2 of this word in the *Middle English Dictionary* (hereafter *M.E.D.*), ed. H. Kurath and S.M. Kuhn, s.v. *bre* is "water of the sea," and an extension of this sense to any kind of saltwater is a possibility. The plural, therefore, could mean waters, urines, or urinations.

64

colour & smellyth* somewhat. But yf withholdyng be of a colde, drye humour that is in her veynes & is cleped melancolye they fele moche hevynesse benetheforth, & her vryn is discoloured & thynne & hathe in hym small gravell otherwhiles of þe colour, as it were, axen and otherwhile the vryn is blak & fatt & theryn be litel blake motes & derke. And in tyme of her purgacion, yf they delyuer hem of ony thyng, it is but litell in quantyte. And women that ben ystopped contynuelly her vryne is medled with litell small thynges as blak as coles; otherwhiles, it is whyt & thykke & derk as mylk; otherwhiles, it is whyt & thynne and whiȝt swamous mater hangyng in þe vryne; other[whiles] small bodyes blak ymedled with þe vryne.

Ther ben corupte humours in þe moder with outen the veynes in the holownesse of þe moder & they letten women of her purgacions. And thre humours ther ben that ben wonte to be in þe moder as fleume, colre, & melancolye. The tokens of fleume be these: they fele moche moystnesse & they haue no lykyng to medle with men. And they fele hevynesse & cold [f. 196v] from the navell dounward and whan thei haue her purgacion thei ben deliuered of moche flewme with þe blode þat þei ben ypurged of. And her vryne is whyt or moche drawyng to whyt. And yf suche humours ben resolued into wynd, þei fle vp to þe hert & to þe longes & make þe woman fle into a cardiacle. But yf þer be moche melancolie in þe moder, þei haue litell likyng to medle with men & whan þei do so þer passith litell mater from hem & they felen moche colde & hevynesse bynethe her navel. And they felen, as it wer, a colde wynde mevyng in þe moder & in þe tyme of her purgacion they ben deliuered of lytell matere and that is medled with melancolye that is of swart yelowe colour, and þe mouthe of the marice, that is to say, herr prevy membre, is astonyed and hathe but litell felyng ne but litell likyng thawgh they medle with men. And her vryne is otherwhiles swart yelowe & fatty & otherwhiles it is [thynne]† & of feble colour. And yf ther be moche colre in þe moder, they fele hete þerin & ache & prykkyng & hardenesse. And they be hoot about þe mouth of þe marice and haven gret desyre & lykyng to company with men & sone they deliuere hem of mater but þe mater is but litell in quantite. And in tyme of her purgacion, yf they be deliuered of ony blood, it ne is but litell & of a rede swart colour.

*smellyth: MS. swellyth.
† [thynne]: MS. ¶.

color and smell slightly. But if the retention is of a cold, dry humor that is in their veins and is called melancholy, women feel much heaviness below, and their urine is discolored, thin, and contains in it some small gravel,* sometimes of the color of ashes, and sometimes the urine is black and greasy, with small black spots, and murky. And during the time of their purgation, if they discharge anything, it is very little in quantity. And in women that are continually stopped up, their urine is mixed with tiny things as black as coals; sometimes it is white, thick, and opaque as milk; other times it is white and thin, and white scaly matter hangs in the urine; sometimes there are small black bodies mixed with the urine.

There are corrupt humors in the womb outside the veins in the hollowness of the uterus, and they hinder women in their purgations. And there are three humors that occur in the uterus, such as phlegm, bile, and black bile. The signs of phlegm are these: women feel much humidity and have no desire to consort with men. And they feel heaviness and coldness [f. 196v] from the navel downward, and when they have their purgation they excrete much phlegm with the blood. And their urine is white or very much tending to white. And if such humors turn into wind, they fly up to the heart and lungs and cause a heart attack. And if there is much black bile in the uterus, women have little desire to consort with men, and when they do so little matter comes from them, and they feel much cold and heaviness below the navel. And they feel as if a cold wind is moving in the uterus, and at the time of their purgation they lose little, and what there is is mingled with black bile that is dark yellow in color, and the mouth of the marice, that is to say, their privy member, is numbed and has little feeling and little pleasure, even though the women consort with men. And their urine is sometimes dark yellow and greasy, and sometimes it is thin and of poor color. And if there is much bile in the uterus, they feel heat inside and aching, pricking, and hardness. And such women feel hot about the mouth of the womb and have great need and liking to go with men, and straightaway they have a discharge, but it is very small. And at the time of their purgation, if they discharge any blood, it is very little and of dark red color.

* See *M.E.D.*, s.v. *gravel* n (c) med. Small concretions of calculous matter in the urine.

*Cura*: For to helpe women of these sekenesses ther be many diuerse medecynes as blode letyng in other places to deliuere hem of blode that they mowe nought ben yporged of & that is profitable lest they falle into a cardiacle oþer into a dropsye. And profitable bledynges ben att þe vyenes of þe gret toon & to be [f. 197r] ygarsed on þe leggis bynethe the sparlyuer bothe byfore & behynd, and to be cupped bynethe þe tetes, & also bynethe þe reynes behynde. Also Stuphes ben profitable to hem ymade of herbes þat wyl & mowe open þe veynes of þe moder þat þe bloode may haue the rather his issue. And yf þei be stopped thorough colre, that is to say, thorough an humour that is hote & drye, late make a stewe of herbes þat ben openyng, as of pollipodie, lorell leves, ivy, savyn, madir, origanum, rosemarie, comyn, affodille,* fenel, mogwede, calamynt, isop, puliole, nept & suche oþer, & lete hir sitte on an holowe stole ouer þese herbis whan they ben wel ysoden & hote. And sythen let hyr drynk a drawȝt of wyne þat mogwede & polipodie ben soden yn & otherwhiles lete make hyr right sorye & oþerwhiles riȝt wrothe & oþerwhiles ryȝt mery & late hyr vsen hote saucis and kene as garlyk & peper & mustard & kersis & suche other & lete bathe hyre in þe bathys ymade of suche herbis as yspake of riȝt nowȝ. And lete hyre walke moche & trauayle wel & ete wele & drynk well, & then they schull liȝtly be purged of hyr blood. And aboute þat tyme of þe mone þat þey schul haue her purgacion, yf they haue noon, lete hem blede a good quantite of blode at her gret too & another day her other gret too. And euerich weke, onys, lete hyre vsen to ben ybathed in suche herbes as I spake of rather, & sche may be holpen though hyr syknes haue dured hir longe tyme. But yf this greuaunce be of cold, first yeve her this medecyne to make the mater that grevith her þe more able to passe lyȝtly awey from hyre.

Take radyche of fe-[f. 197v] nell, parcely, dawk and merche, the rotes of these & nouȝt þe leves, & then take the leves of mogwede, of savyne, of calament, of origanum—yef thou hast nouht alle these herbes, take tho that þou mayst come to—& sethe hem in vyneger for to they be wel ysoden; & then clense hit & caste to the vynegre halfe so moche honye as the vynegre is & lete hem two boyle togeder a whyle ouer the fyre, & sithen, whan it is colde, lete hir vsen therof a two dayes or thre but medle it with water that radices and madir ben sothen yn.

*affodile: MS. offodille.

*Cure*: To help women in these illnesses there are various remedies, such as blood-letting in other places to get rid of the blood that they cannot be cleansed of, and this is useful in case they may suffer heart disease or dropsy. And useful bleedings are at the veins of the big toe and [f. 197r] cuts on the legs below the calf, both in front and behind, and cupping under the nipples and also under the kidneys at the back. Also baths are useful to them, made from herbs able to open the veins of the uterus so that the blood can emerge more quickly. And if the stoppage is due to bile, that is to say, through a humor that is hot and dry, have made a hot bath of seasonal herbs that are aperients, such as polypody, laurel leaves, ivy, savin, madder, origanum, rosemary, cumin, asphodel, fennel, artemisia, calamint, hyssop, wild thyme, catmint, and such other herbs, and let her sit on a hollow stool over these herbs when they are well boiled and hot. And afterward let her drink a draught of wine in which artemisia and polypody are boiled and sometimes cause her to be very unhappy, sometimes very angry, sometimes very merry, and let her use hot and piquant relishes such as garlic, pepper, mustard, cresses, and other such things, and let her bathe in baths made from such herbs as I have just spoken of. And let her walk a great deal, work, eat and drink well, and then she will be easily purged of her blood. And about that time of the moon that women should have their purgation, if they have none, have them bled a considerable quantity of blood at their big toe one day, and another day at their other big toe. And once every week accustom the woman to take a bath in such herbs as I spoke of earlier, and she may be helped even though her sickness has lasted a long time. But if the complaint is of a cold humor, first give her this medicine to make it more possible for her trouble to pass easily away from her.

Take fe-[f. 197v]nnel root, parsley, wild carrot, celery, the roots of these and not the leaves, and then take the leaves of artemisia, savin, calamint, origanum—if you don't have all these herbs take what you have—and cook them in vinegar so that they are well boiled; and then clean the mixture, throw into the vinegar half as much honey as there is vinegar, boil the two together for a time over the fire, and afterward, when it is cold, let her use it two or three days mixed with water in which radishes and madder have been boiled.

And after that, lete stue here and bathen hyr with suche herbes as I sayd rather & after þat this is sodden, lete hyr drynk a drauȝt of wyne that savyne other mogwode other madir is soden yn & medle that wyne with water that polipodie is soden in. And yf they haue no purgacion, lete hem blede a good quantite of blode as I sayd afore. Suppositories* ben couenable medecynes for these sykenesses. And they schul be putte in womens prevy membres as men putteth suppositories into a mannes fundement for to purgen his wombe. But these suppositories that ben ordeyned for women schuld be bounde with a threde abouten oon of her thyes lest they were drawe all into þe moder. And it is profitable to vsen suche suppositories a foure dayes other a fyve before that tyme of þe moneth that they schull haue her purgacion & they mowe the liȝtlyer ben ypurged. On suppositorie is this: Take triacle diatesseron 3 *sem.* and of cocle floure as moche & as moche of mirre, & stampe hem togeder with boles galle þat savyn or rewe is rotened withyn; then make hit vp with cotton & therof make a suppositorie as gret as thy litell fynger and putte in her prevy membre [f. 198r]. But anoynte it first with clene hony and oyle togeder and strewe þeron pouder of skamony, & put in þe prevy membre; thus myȝt a man do with the rote of lupines & that is moche better. Another supposytorye: Take the rote of smallache—the mountance of thy fynger—all grene, & larde hit with the rote of pileter of Spayne & sithen putt that rote in þe erth ayen a fourtenyght or a thre wekys and than take it vp and wipe hit clene and putte it into her prevy membre all day and all a nyght; and afterward take it owt and anoynte it with oyle of lorer oþer with mete oile & putt it in eftsones, and lete it ligge till sche haue here purgacion. For though ther were a dede chylde in her wombe it wolde brynge it ouȝt. And þe same virtue hathe the rote of actory† & also best is the rotis of vyns yf it be diȝt in the same wyse. But or than sche vnderfonge this suppositorie, thou schalt sethe savyne & fursis, puliol! riall, lorer leues in water & lete þe woman sitte þerin a good whyle afterward and sithen lete her wasshe hir prevy membre as depe as sche may reche inward & thus do a good whyle with water; then do drye her with a clothe & putt in þat suppositorie of apium or of acorns vt supra.

*MS. margin: *Suppositorie.*

†i.e., accory. Common variant spellings will be noted only when their presence interferes with the sense.

And after that, let her soak and bathe herself in such herbs as
I referred to earlier, and when the mixture is cooked let her
drink a draught of wine in which savin, artemisia, or madder is
boiled in, and mix that wine with water that polypody is boiled
in. And if women have no purgation, let them bleed a good
quantity of blood, as I said previously. Suppositories are useful
medicines for these maladies. And they should be put in a
woman's privy member just as a man puts a suppository in his
anus in order to cleanse his stomach. But these suppositories for
women should be fastened with a thread* bound round one of
her thighs, in case the suppositories should be drawn
completely into the uterus. And it is a good thing to use such
suppositories four or five days before the time of the month
when women have their purgation, to make it easier. One
suppository is this: take half a drachm of *triacle diatesseron*,† the
same amounts of cockle flour and myrrh, and grind them
together with bull's gall in which savin or rue has been rotted.
And then cover the mixture with cotton and thereof make a
suppository as large as your little finger and put it in her privy
member. [f. 198r] But first anoint it with clean honey and oil
together, sprinkle powder of scammony on it, and put it in the
privy member; one can do the same with lupin root, and that is
much better. Another suppository: take the root of smallage—
the size of your finger—all green, and grease it with the root of
pellitory of Spain, and afterward put that root in the earth again
for a fortnight or for three weeks, then take it up, wipe it clean,
and put it into her privy member all day and all night; and
afterward take it out, anoint it with oil of laurel or with a
suitable oil, put it in again, and let it remain there until she has
her purgation. For even if there was a dead child in her womb, it
would bring it out. And the root of yellow iris has the same
virtue, and vine roots, if prepared in the same way, are also
excellent. But before she receives this suppository you must boil
savin, furze, pennyroyal, laurel leaves in water, and have the
woman sit in the water for a considerable time afterward, and
then have her wash her privy member as far in as she can do,
and do so for a good while; then dry her with a cloth and put in
that suppository of wild celery or of acorns, as above.

* A kind of medieval tampon.
† A medicament with four ingredients.

Another suppositorie*: Take þe floure of cokell and medle hit with hony & with coton & make a suppositorie therof.

Anoþer is this: Take peleter of Spayne ʒ iii, of litell peleter as moche, cokell flour ʒ i, of diagredii ʒ vii, putte all these into a litell lynnen bagge that thy fynger wold in & lete hyr putt it in as depe as sche may so þat sche may pullen hit oute liʒtlich, for it wyl make hyre haue a purgacion anone. Yef her wombe be sore of suche suppositories [f. 198v], lete anoynte withyn with oyle of roses or of violet or with mete oile or with fresshe butter þat is not salted. Other medecynes ther ben the whiche yf a woman drynk hem they wyl make hyre to haue a purgacion other deliver hir of a dede chyld yf þer be ony withyn hire, as bawme precious ydronk and þe jus of isop, other of diptayn & of leke & of tounkers & þe seed of tounkers ypouderd and ydronken. But yf þis siknesse come of angre other of sorowe, lete mak hir mery & yeve hyre comfortable metes and drynkes and lete vsyn hyr to bathen hyre otherwhiles. And yf it be of moche fastyng oþer of moche wakyng, lete diete hyr moche with good metes and drynkes that mowe make hyr to haue good blode, & lete hyr make hyr mery and glade & leven þe hevinesse of her hevy þoughtes.

Good electuaries† for this sekenesse ben Theodoricon enperi-con, theodoricon anacardi, & trifera magna, panchristum,‡ and diaspermaton is þe beste of hem alle.

Also a worschipfull serip þat myʒtyly bringeth forth the corupt blode fro þe moder & this seryp is for ladyes & for nunnes & other also þat ben delicate. $R_x$: rotes of litell madir, knowholme, sparage rotes, & þe rote of ciperi ana quartern *sem.*, of mogwede; of savyne, nept,§ valerian, calament, puliole ana *m.* i, herbe baume *m.* ii, the seed of sermontayne ʒ i, spikenard ʒ *sem.*, misid, liquorice, reysons and her stones ypyked out ana ʒ i, the floures & þe leves grene of rosemary, floures of sticados arabice ana ʒ i, clene hony *li. sem.*, of lofe sugre quartern iii; make a sirup yclarified *li.* i & *sem.* and yeve to þe women two ounces

*MS. margin: *Suppositorie.*
† MS. margin: *Electuars.*
‡ magna, panchristum,: MS. magnum paxum.
§ nept: MS. next.

Another suppository: take cockle flour and mix it with honey and with cotton and make a suppository of it.

Another one is: take 3 drachms of pellitory of Spain, the same amount of little pellitory, 1 drachm of cockle flour, 7 drachms of scammony. Put all these in a small linen bag that your finger would go in, and let her put it in as far as she can if she is to pull it out again easily, because this will cause her to have a purgation right away. If her womb is sore as a result of such suppositories, [f. 198v] have her anointed inside with oil of roses or violet or with a suitable oil or with fresh unsalted butter. There are other medicines that, if drunk, will cause a woman to have a purgation or abort a dead child if there is one inside her, such as precious balm drunk, and the juice of hyssop or dittany, leeks, nasturtiums, and nasturtium seed, powdered and drunk. But if this illness is a result of anger or sorrow, cause her to be cheerful, give her refreshing food and drink, and get her used to bathing herself sometimes. And if it is the result of much fasting or overwakefulness, see that she eats good food and drink which will give her good blood, and get her to enjoy herself and be happy and give up gloomy thoughts.

Good medical cordials for this sickness are theodoricon empiricon, theodoricon anacardinum,* trifera† magna, panchristum,‡ and diaspermaton is the best of all. Also, a good syrup that is very effective in bringing out corrupt blood from the uterus, and it is for ladies, nuns, and other women who are delicate. Take half a measure § each of roots of little madder, butcher's-broom, asparagus, and the root of galingale, 1 handful each of artemisia, savin, catmint, valerian, calamint, and thyme, 2 handfuls of herb balsam, 1 ounce of the seed of mountain willow, half an ounce of spikenard mixed, 1 drachm of licorice, stoned raisins, the flowers and green leaves of rosemary, and flowers of Arabian sticados, half a pound of clean honey, 3 measures of loaf sugar; make 1½ pounds of clarified syrup, and give the women either 2 ounces

---

* Theodoricons are ordinary purgatives; theodoricon anacardi is an antidote for cold ailments of the head—called *theodoricon* because it is a gift of God and *anacardinum* because made from an apple that is heart-shaped. Theodoricon Empiricon is a purgative tested by experience and found to be effective (*empiricon*).

† Trifera (trypheron) is a mild purgative made from plums and good for the stomach.

‡ Panchristum: "useful for everything," was known to Pliny as a mouthwash made from mulberries (*NH*, XXIII, 136–38).

§ Quartern: a quarter of a specified weight.

þerof & oþer two of þe decoction of rede chiches, oþer do þerto *li*. iiii fyne clarre, other of fyne pyment, and do to þe serup & [f. 199r] medle hem wel togeder and yeve hyr þerof erlych and late, at euery tyme ʒ vi & yeve hyr ʒ ii of benedicte in hir potage and make hir potage hereof: Take* fenell leves, avens, borage, violet, watercrassen, stanmarche, isop, saueray, mercurie, malues, chervile ana ʒ ii and make wortes and lete hir ete oon messe grene with benedicta ʒ i, and another messe more ysoden with benedicta ʒ i, & it is esy; and yf thou yeve hyr drynk of hit clere made with þe serup a gret drawʒt and it schal purgen bothe the marice & also þe body esilich; and withouten penaunce to do this in a cloos chambre from colde & from eyre. Also to make a pelewe† that þe women schulde sitte on whiles thei ben in the stuphe for to mollifie harde retencions & to nesshen þe weyes of þe marice ys thus made: Take mogwede, of saueray ana *m*. ii, the leves of pastinake, þe leves of costi, of malues, marsshmalowe, lynesede, fenugreke, of doder, hempsed, lauender, sede of sermountayne ana ʒ ii, persely sede, fenel sede, anisi, anete, asari, dauci ana ʒ *sem.*, floures of camomille, floures of elleryn, of rosmaryn, of bothe sticudos ana ʒ ii, al to bete hem in a mortar & putte hem into a poket litell—to þe quantite of a span brode & in length; whan this bagge is fulled, lete þe woman sitte þeron in þe bath. And whan sche comyth out of þe bath, late anoynte here with oyle myscelyn þe whiche is wreten in þe chapiter off suffocacion herafterward. And yeve her to drynk electuarie hemagoge‡ ʒ ii with wyne þat archime is soden yn or panchristum with meche & lete bryngen hyre in a bedde riʒt esely made. And then yeve hir a suppositorie prouocatyf. Item: Take isope rotes, [f. 199v] of gladon, of savyne, of rue, of saueray ana ʒ iiii, of diptayn, of nept, of fenell sede, of ameos sede ana ʒ ii, whiʒt wyne of Gascoyne *li*. i & *sem.*, of clene rennyng water *li*. i, of mirre Ꝺ vii; & bray thy sedes and stampe thyne herbes and þe mirr riʒt small & lete sethe hem a while & lete it

*MS. margin: *Laxatyff*.
† MS. margin: *Pelow*.
‡ hemagoge: MS. emagoge.

of this or 2 ounces of a stew of red chick-peas, or add to it 4
pounds of fine claret or fine spice, add it to the syrup, [f. 199r]
mix the ingredients well together, give them to her at all hours,
6 ounces every time, and give her 2 ounces of benedicta* in her
soup, and make her soup of the following: take 2 ounces each of
fennel leaves, avens, borage, violets, watercress, horse-parsley,
hyssop, savory, mercury,† mallows, chervil, and make pottage,
and let her eat one portion green with 1 drachm of benedicta,
and another portion further cooked with 1 drachm of benedicta,
and it is satisfying. And if you give her to drink a big draught of
it entirely made with the syrup, it will easily purge both the
womb and the body; and to avoid suffering do this in a room that
is secluded from cold and draft. Also, here is a prescription for a
pillow that women should sit on while they are in the bath in
order to reduce painful retentions and soften the processes of
the womb. Take 2 handfuls each of artemisia, savory, 2 drachms
each of parsnip leaves, costmary leaves, mallows, marshmallows,‡ linseed, fenugreek, flax dodder, hempseed, lavender,
mountain willow seed, half a drachm each of parsley seed, fennel seed, anise, dill, hazelwort, wild carrots, 2 drachms each
of camomile flowers, sambucus flowers, rosemary, both kinds
of sticados, beat them all together in a mortar and put them in
a little bag—the size of a span in breadth and length: when this
bag is filled let the woman sit on it in the bath. And when she
comes out of the bath have her anointed with musk oil, which is
described in the chapter concerning suffocation later on. And
give her to drink 2 drachms of hemagogue§ electuary with wine
that mugwort is boiled in or panchristum with *meche*,** and have
her brought into a comfortably made bed. And then give her a
stimulating suppository. Take 4 drachms each of hyssop roots,
[f. 199v] iris, savin, rue, savory, 2 drachms each of dittany, catmint, fennel seed, seed of bishop's-weed, 1½ pounds of white
wine of Gascony, 1 pound of clean running water, 7 scruples of
myrrh; crush your seeds, pound your herbs and the myrrh
extremely small, and boil them for awhile, and then let

* An electuary used in various medicines.
† Herb, variously identified in the *Oxford English Dictionary* [hereafter O.E.D.]
and M.E.D., probably dog's foot (*mercurialis perennis*).
‡ The European herb marshmallow (*Althaea officinalis*).
§ A cordial-like medicament used to draw out the blood.
** M.E.D. s.v. *mecche* n. gives (a) the wick of a candle or lamp; (b) *surg.* = lich-
ine. A plug, sometimes impregnated with a medicament.

stonde til it be cold; clense hit as moch as sche may drynke at onys by þe morewe. Also yeve it with trociskys of deliueryng of chyld that ben wreten in þe chapiter of mola matricis with other medecynes and plasters ther ywreten. And thys medecyn bothe bryngeth forth dede chyld & quyke whereuer it be in þe womans wombe & þat sone. Also this emplaster solutyf, yef it be layd on a womannys schare, it deliuereth a dede chyld oþer of ony other best þer ybredde, & yf it be leyd on þe stomak it makith her to spewe. And yf it be leid on þe wombe it makith her to go to prevy. R$_x$ electuarie ii, elibori nigri ana ʒ iiii, lattide* ʒ iii, ciclaminis† interioris, colloquitide, succi, titumalle ana ʒ 6, cocanidii ʒ ii, turbentini ʒ iiii, melli quod sufficit. But I, forsothe, do to this medecyn in þe stede of hony galbanum li. sem. whan it schal do it to deliuere a woman from hir chyld. And yf I shal make a laxatyf, I putte þerto May butter þat is fressh with a good quantite of boles gall.

*The secunde chapiter is of to moche flowyng of blode in vntyme; and this sikenesse febleth moche women.*

To moche flowyng of blode at þis membre comyth in many maners: as of gret plente of blode that is in þe woman; other it is of þe kenesse of þe blode þat þorugh his keneschip perissheth veynes; other it is of þe sotilte of þe blode þat swetith out þorugh þe small [f. 200r] porys of the veynes & so flowith oute; other for the blode is vndefied and rennyng & thynne as water; other it is of feblenesse of þe woman that may not withholden þe blode withyn hyre; other it is for some brekyng of some veyne þat is in þe prevy membre oþer ther nygh.
Yef it be in þe first maner, they bledyn & they felen hete & smertyng in her prevy membre and they be deliuered of to litell bloode and that comyth swyftly forthe oute; and oþer yt is blak or yelow as safran or of þe coloure of fyre. And they haue otherwhile her gomes ycloue and her nether lippes of her mouth and they fele smertyng and akyng & prikkyng aboute her tetes. And but yf it be in þe third maner, the blode comyth softli a litell & a litell & þat is thynne & clere. And yf it is of hete, he schall fynde hete withynforth & oþer tokens of hete withynforth & withouten. And yf it is of the ferth maner, þe blode is watery & thynne, and sche hathe euyll defying bothe in here stomak & in

---

*lattide. Presumably lactuce is meant.
† ciclaminis: MS. ciclamie.

them stand until cold; strain as much as she is likely to drink at one time by the morning. Also give it with pills for delivering the child that are described in the chapter of *mola matricis* along with other medicines and plasters. And this medicine both brings forth a dead child and a live child wherever it is in the woman's womb and that forthwith. Also this relaxing plaster, if it is laid on a woman's genitals, delivers a dead child or any other creature* that grows there, and if it is laid on the stomach, it makes her throw up. And if it is laid on the womb, it makes her go to the privy. Take 2 drachms of electuary, 4 drachms of black hellebore, 3 drachms of lettuce, 6 ounces each of the inside of the cyclamen, colocynth juice, spurge, 2 of laurel seeds, 4 of terebinth resin, honey as suffices. But I, to tell the truth, add half a pound of galbanum to this medicine instead of honey when it is to make a woman give birth. And if I want to make a laxative, I add to it May butter that is fresh, with a good quantity of bull's gall.

*The second chapter is concerned with excessive flowing of blood at the wrong time; and this sickness weakens a great number of women.*

Excessive discharge of blood at the vagina comes in many ways: through the great amount of blood that is in the woman; or through the fierceness of the blood that through its strength destroys veins; or through the thinness of the blood that sweats out through the small [f. 200r] pores of the veins and so flows out; or through the blood being undigested and runny and thin as water; or through the weakness of the woman who cannot keep the blood inside her; or through the breaking of some vein that is in the privy member or near to it.

If the discharge is in the first way, they bleed and feel heat and smarting in their privy member, and they lose very little blood, and it comes out quickly; or it is black or yellow as saffron or the color of fire. And they sometimes have their gums stuck together and the lower lip of the mouth, and they feel a smarting, aching, and pricking about the nipples. And if it is in the third way, the blood comes gently, little by little, and is thin and clear. And if the discharge is from heat, one will find heat inside and other signs of heat inside and out. And if it is in the fourth way, the blood is watery and thin, and she has bad digestion both in her stomach and in

* Meaning a fetus in the early stages of development.

her wombe & sche felith hurlyng wyndes vp & down in hir wombe. And yf it be in þe fyft manere, thow myght knowe it by the feblenesse of þe womans body; and þe blode þat passith from hyre it comyth febelych & contynually, and in his goyng it makith noon anguysshe ne greuaunce. And yf it be in þe sixt manere, the blode comyth contynually & with greuaunce, and oþerwhile it hath his kyndely coloure and oþerwhiles it hathe nought but comyth out corrupt in maner of quyttour. And whereof euer this siknesse comyth and in what manere, þou schall nouȝt sodenly stoppe þe blode of his flowyng ne none maner of fluxe but yf a man oþer a woman be þe more yfeblyd [f. 200v] therby, for than man schull sesen it as sone as men may and ellis nouȝt.

*Cura*: And yf þer come grete plenty of blode, lete dryen her with metes & drynkes that gendryn but litell blode,* as frute & herbes & lete hyr blede at þe veyne of hir arme and to be cupped vnder hyr tetes and abouten þe reynes & the lendes, and to be garsed on her legges to withdrawen the blode awaywardis from þe moder.

A powder† : Take psidia, ypoquistides, acasia, colophonia & make þerof suppositories or medle all these with þe jus of planteyne & enplastre it aboute bothe before on þe moder & behynde even ayenst hit. Oþer medecyns also þat be good to staunche þe blodye fluxe: as take a gret rote of Enule campane *li. sem*. & ℥ vi, of clene water a galon & a half; sethe hem to a potell & than clense it & putt þerto half a *li*. of whyte sugre & sethe it eftsones a litell & lete hyt cele. And lete here drynke þerof erliche & late & hit schall staunche withyn iiii dayes; this medecyne taught þe Pryor of Bermondesey to a woman þat was nygh dede on þe fluxe of hyre marice. And to amende hyr stomak, he lete take two handful of þe medell rynde of þe brome & lete sethe hyt in thre potell of clere water to a potell; clense hit & putt þerto a half a *li*. of whyt suger & lete sethe eftsones & yef hyr to drynke. But yf this fluxe come of a lennes and of a scharpnesse‡ of þe blode, lete her bleden a litell on þe arme & sithen lete hyr drynke a litell rubarbe§ ℥ ii, sene ℥ ii, with þe jus cocte, & borage & fenell ana ℥ vi, to make her blode clene, & sithen lete hyre drynke þe jus of mente & of popy & of planteyne, clarified and skymede, & [f. 201r] that wyl staunche þe bledynge. And yf þou do þerto þe jus

*MS. margin: *Of to moche bloode.*
† MS. margin: *Suppositorie.*
‡ MS. margin: *Of sharpnesse.*
§ rubarb: MS. rubarke.

her womb, and she feels winds rumbling up and down in her womb. And if it is in the fifth way, you can tell by the weakness of the woman's body; and the blood that comes from her is scanty and continuous, and its passing causes neither distress nor pain. And if it is in the sixth way, the blood comes continuously and with pain, and sometimes it has its natural color, sometimes it has none but comes out impaired in the manner of pus. And wherever the sickness comes from and in what way, you cannot suddenly stop the flowing of blood nor any kind of flux unless a man or woman is further weakened [f. 200v] thereby; therefore, one can only stop it as quickly as one can and nothing else.

*Cure*: And if there is a great quantity of blood, dehydrate her with food and drink that produce only a little blood, such as fruit and herbs, and have her bled at the vein of her arm and be cupped under her nipples and about the kidneys and loins, and scarified on her legs to draw the blood away from the uterus.

A powder: take pomegranate, hypocistis,* acacia, colophony, and make suppositories of them, or mix all these with the juice of plantain and plaster it both in front of the womb and behind it and even in contact with it. Other medicines that are also good to staunch the bloody flux: take a great root of horseheal—half a pound and 6 ounces, 1½ gallons of clean water; boil them to a pottle,† strain it, add half a pound of white sugar, boil it again for a while, and let it cool. And let her drink it at all hours, and it will stop the blood within four days; the Prior of Bermondesey taught this medicine to a woman who was almost dead from the flux in her womb. And to cure her stomach he prescribed: take 2 handfuls of the center rind of broom and let it boil in 3 pottles of clear water to a pottle; strain it, add to it half a pound of white sugar, let the mixture boil afterward, and give it her to drink. But if this flux is due to emaciation and fierceness of the blood, have her bled a little on the arm and afterward let her drink a little rhubarb—2 drachms, 2 drachms of senna boiled with the liquid, and 6 ounces each of borage and fennel to cleanse her blood, and afterward let her drink the juice of mint, poppy, plantain clarified and skimmed, and [f. 201r] that will staunch the bleeding. And if you add to the mixture the juice of the daisy and powder of oak gall used in

* See *M.E.D.* s.v. *ipoquistidos.*
† Half a gallon.

of þe daysye and þe pouder of galles, þat men make ynke of, it wyl sownden & helen þe veynes that be broken thorough scharpnesse of þat blode; & lete here vsen hokkes, betes, violettis, planteyne in her potage to abaten þe kenes of þe blode, & let hyr vsen porselane, letuse, mente, planteyne, sorell & roses in medecyns to make þe flux to sese. Also let hyr vsen comfery & daysye ana ℥ i. R$_x$: gallie, sangdragon, bole, corallis albi & rubie, manne masticis ana ℈ ii, conserue rosarum ℥ ii, zucari albi ℥ v teranda & conficiantur. And lete her vsen this electuarie with þe jus off planteyn or moleyne; or ellis take þis same pouder & sethe it in rayne water & make a pissarie & so minister her with. This wyl sowde þe veynes that ben broke. Also take ceruse, almandes, muscillage of psillii ana ℥ i & *sem.*, lete wetyn a weke therin & putte it in her prevy membre in manere of a suppositorie. Also a plaster made of muscillage of psillium, of lynesede ypoudred, of dragaunce yleyde on her schare, it is profitable for þis greuaunces. Also take þe pouder of psillium ybrand & gipsum ybrand & bole & sandar, psidie, acornys of okes, balaustia or in stede of it þe oken ryndes & symphite & sumak ana ℥ ii & *sem.*, camphore ℥ i *sem.*; poudre alle these in fere & temper it with whyte of eyren & make two enplasters þerof— oon to lye on þe schare & another to lye on þe reynes. And this maladie comyth of þe succide* of þe blode, lete her usen comfortabyl electuaries. And namely yf a woman be of feble complexion, Athanasie ℥ ii, succari albi rosarum ℥ *sem.*, diacitoniten, diacodion, gallie muscillage ana ℥† 12 & *sem.*, zucari albi [f. 201v] ℥ v cum succo plantaginis in quo lapis ematites fuerit fricatus, and lete diete her with metes that wyl make her blode thikke, as with almaunde mylk & ryse made with almaunde mylk and furmentye. Also menge therwith gotes mylk for that is full profitable for this syknesse for it makith þe blode thyk & sowdith the veynes þat ben broken & letted the blode of his flowyng. But for to make hyt riȝt profitable, take clene stones þat haue longe leyen in clene rennyng water & hete hem well in the fyre & sithen quenche hem in þe mylk of almaundes, in þe mylk of a gote that is fedde with good herbes, or with cowes

*MS. margin: *Of suscite of bloode.*
† The ounce sign here is a scilicet sign, not repeated in this text.

making ink, the medicine will make whole and heal the veins that are broken because of the fierceness of the blood; and let her use mallows, beets, violets, plantain in her soup to reduce the fierceness of the blood, and purslane, lettuce, mint, plantain, sorrel, and roses in medicines to stop the flux. Also let her use 1 drachm each of comfrey and daisy. Prescription: grind 2 scruples each of gall, sandragon, Armenian bole,* white and red coral, gum of mastic, 2 drachms of conserve of roses, 5 drachms of white sugar, and have them put together. And let her use this electuary with the juice of plantain or mullein; or else take this same powder, boil it in rainwater, make a pessary, and so give it to her. This will heal the veins that are broken. Also take 1½ ounces each of white lead, almonds, the juice from fleawort, moisten a wick in it and put it in her privy member in the manner of a suppository. Also a plaster made of juice of fleawort, powdered linseed, dragonwort placed on her genitals is profitable for these disorders. Also take the powder of burnt fleawort, burnt gypsum, Armenian bole, sandalwood, pomegranate, oak acorns, flowers of wild pomegranate or in place of them 2 drachms each of oak rinds, wallwort, and sumac, 1 drachms of camphor; powder these all together, mix white of egg with the decoction, and make two plasters of it, one to lie on the genitals and another on the kidneys. And should this malady be due to the cutting off of blood, let her use comforting electuaries. And especially if the woman is of feeble complexion, 2 drachms of Athanasia,† half an ounce of white sugar of roses, 12 ounces each of diacitonicon syrup, diacodion syrup,‡ mucilage of oak gall, 5 drachms of white sugar [f. 201v] with juice of plantain in which hematite has been rubbed, and let her have a diet of food that will thicken her blood, such as almond milk, rice made with almond milk, and frumenty.§ Also mix with goat's milk, for it is excellent for this illness because it makes the blood thick and heals the veins that are broken and hinder the flowing of blood. To make the medication really efficacious, take clean stones that have been for a long time in clean running water, heat them well in the fire, and afterward cool them in the almond milk, in the milk of a goat that has been fed with good herbs, or with cow's

* A red astringent earth.
† A compound medicine.
‡ For these two syrups, see *M.E.D.* s.v. *dia-* (a).
§ A pottage of boiled, hulled grain, sweetened and mixed with milk or almond milk.

mylk, and they schall consume þe watrynesse of þe mylk, and lete her vsen good moton and good hennes that ben wel flesshyd and litell fatte. And amonge all thyngis that men vsen, rys and whete thikkith moche a mannes blode, and wortes made of arage & of betes makith blode thynne. And lete her vsen zucarum rosarum & diapapa[ve]re, & these pillen lete her vsen whan sche gothe to bedde & erlich whan sche arisith. Take munne, olibani, mastik, & the hertys horne ybrent till it be whyʒt, & of eueriche of these lyche moche, & pouder hem, & tempere hem with the jus of mynte other of planteyne or of mugwede & make hem of the quantite of a bene & lete hyre vsen two other þre at one tyme. And yf þou takyst þe mawe of a soking hare or of a sokyng calf & doyst brenne it to pouder & medelist with þe pouder aforesaid with þe pillis foresaid, they wyl be moche þe better. Also take hertys hornes wel ybrent 3 *sem.*, of eyshelles ¼ iii, poudre all these thre togeder and lete her vsen it in potage [f. 202r], in sawce, and in drynk; probatum est in Chepa, London.
Another:* Take lynesede al hole and sethe it in schepis mylk oþer gotys mylk & lete her ete it, other fenugrek, þat is moche better. Take þe rotes of dragaunce 3 v, the leves of merche 3 iii, pouder these in fere & drynk it with good ale, and sche shal be hole; this was provyd at Surcester on Barons wyf þat was nygh dede on this maladie.* Another: Also þe jus of mugwede ydronk, oþer þe herbe yplasterd is gode to staunche the fluxe. And yf this syk-nesse come of feblenesse of a womans complexion,† lete here vsen confortable metes and drynkes, and zucarum rosarum and diapapa[ve]re, and þe jus of myntes yclarified & sothen & caste þerto a litell quantite of sugre to make hit swete. Another: Take encense, mente, sangdragon & mastik & violet & storax, rubie ana 3 vi; pouder all these in fere with þe jus of planteyne & with vyneger & plastre‡ hit bothe before & behynde, id est, on hyre share & on hyr reynes. And yf it come of brekyng of veynes,§ the foresaid suppositories & electuaries be good for hem. And oþer medecyns ther ben ful good that staunche the blody fluxe & they be good for þis sykenesse. And to take a fat ele & ley hym al quyk on þe koles, and lete þe woman stonde þerouer & lete þe smoke

*Repeated and dotted for expunction.
† MS. margin: *Feblenesse of compleccion*.
‡ plastre: MS. pastre.
§ MS. margin: *Of brekyng of veynes*.

milk, and they will absorb the wateriness of the milk, and have her eat juicy mutton and plump hens that are well covered in meat and have little fat. And among all the things that people use, rice and wheat very much thicken the blood, and broth made from orach and beets thins the blood. And let her take sugar of roses and poppy syrup, and let her use these pills when she goes to bed and early when she rises. Take frankincense,* olibanum, mastic, and hartshorn burnt until it is white, and of every one of these a similar amount, powder them, mix them with the juice of mint, plantain, or artemisia, make them the size of a bean, and have her take two or three at a time. And if you take the stomach of a sucking hare or sucking calf, burn it to powder, and mix it with the previously mentioned powder and pills, they will be much better. Also take half a drachm of hartshorn, well burnt, 3 drachms of egg shells, powder all these three† together and let her use it in broth, [f. 202r] in sauce, and in drink; it proved successful in Cheapside, London.

Another: take whole linseed, boil it in sheep's or goat's milk and have her eat it or fenugreek, which is much better. Take 5 drachms of the roots of dragonwort, 3 drachms of the leaves of celery, powder these together, and drink it with good ale, and she will be healed; this was demonstrated at Cirencester on the Baron's wife, who was almost dead from this complaint. Another: the juice of artemisia drunk or made into a plaster is good to staunch the flux. And if this sickness is due to the weakness of a woman's natural constitution, have her take comforting food and drink, sugar of roses, poppy syrup, and the juice of mint strained and boiled with a small quantity of sugar to make it sweet. Another: take 6 drachms each of incense, mint, sandragon, mastic, violets, gum, madder; powder these all together with the juice of plantain and with vinegar, and plaster it both before and behind, that is, on the genitals and kidneys. And if it is the result of veins breaking, the previously mentioned suppositories and electuaries are good for them. And there are other very good medicines that staunch the bloody flux, and they are good for this sickness. Take a fat eel, put it live on the coals, let the woman stand over it, and let the smoke go

* Munne, munnye, manne, maune are all variant spellings for the Latin *manna*: a grain, generally of frankincense (also fols. 201r and 202v). MS. Bodley 178, fol. 154v, remarks that "munna . . . is founden in dede menes graves theras thei ben buryed with precios oynementis."
† The third ingredient is not specified.

come into her prevy membre or into a mannes fundament yef he haue þe fluxe & [f. 202v] in þe same maner do with colophonie. A profitable bathe for this syknesse & also for þe fluxe: Take a good quantite of iren with water & þe fyfte parte þerof stronge vineger & sethe therin þe rynde of þe blak plomtre & of an openerse tre & of a chestayn tre & of an oke, of roses, planteyne, of comfery, the rynde of ayssh, daysye, rybworte, mente, acornys of an oke, pentaphilon smoleynt ysode allone in rede wyne, & plasterd before & behynde shal staunche be his owne myght. But sethe alle these thingis in water tyl þat water be blak and thyk, and lete wrappe þe man oþer þe woman in a shete & sytte in þat bath and lete vsen rosted metes & brede of whete mele made with þe jus of planteyne & of myllefoyle; lete ete partriches yrosted oþer hennes yrosted with wax & lete her vsen to drynke water of roses & of planteyne, oþer ellis reyne water or els water þat mastik is soden in, oþer wyne medled with water. Or els, take water of roses ℥ xviii, masticis ʒ ii, galange ℥ i & *sem.* & Ɵ i, macis, cucube, nardi, cinamoni ana ʒ i; pulverizentur & put all tho into o potte of glasse with þe water of rosarum zuccarum ℥ ii; stop it & lete it sethe in water an houre. This water ydronk is good for all manere syknesse of þe hert in a colde cause & for þe cardiacle & for swownyng & for the fluxe ycome of colde. Also, take a quyk turtille and brenne hyre al quyk with the fetheren, and take an ℥ i of munne & also moche of sangdragon & brenne hem þerwith in an erthyn potte al to poudre. And late her vsen þat poudre in sauce, in potage, & in drynk. Also make pouder of hertis horne ybrente & of eye shelles ybrent ana ℥ x & drynk of þis pouder two drammes at ones with þe jus of planteyne oþer [f. 203r] good mene ale that is not myghty, & she shal staunche. Also take bole armoniak, caruisede ana ʒ iii, zinziber ʒ i, corall fyne and rede ʒ i; make pouder & gyf it hyr and it staunchith. A good medecyne for this maide fluxes: Take galingale, canelle ana ʒ ii, corall rede & þe whyte ana ʒ iii, sangdragon, bole armoniak ana ʒ ii & *sem.*, gum arabici, mirtill coliandri infusi [ʒ] i, prunis albi* & nigri, acasie,† liquorice ana ʒ *sem.*; make pouder herof & gyve it her with þe jus of pervynke, or of planteyne make pouder herof or of turmentill or of roste bones or of molyn. Also take ipoquistidos, acasia,

*albi: MS. al.
† acasie: MS. acusie.

up her privy member, or into a man's anus if he has the flux, and [f. 202v] do the same thing with colophony. A useful bath for this sickness and also for the flux: take a good quantity of iron with water and the fifth part of strong vinegar and boil in it the bark of the black plum tree, a medlar tree, a chestnut tree, an oak, roses, plantain, comfrey, the bark of ash, daisy, ribwort, mint, oak acorns, molemonium* cooked alone in red wine, and [this decoction] plastered before and behind will staunch of its own strength. But boil all these things in water until the water is black and thick, and let the man or woman be wrapped in a sheet and sit in that bath and eat roasted foods and wheat meal bread made with the juice of plantain and milfoil. Have the patient eat roasted partridges or hens roasted in wax, and drink water of roses and plantain, or rainwater or water that mastic is boiled in, or wine mixed with water. Or else take 18 ounces of water of roses, 2 drachms of mastic, 1  ounces and 1 scruple of galingale, 1 drachm each of mace, cucumber, spikenard, cinnamon; have them powdered and put all of them into one glass pot with 2 ounces of water of rose sugar; bottle it and let it boil in water for an hour. This water, if drunk, is good for all kinds of illnesses of the heart due to cold, heart attack, fainting, and for the flux caused by cold. Also, take a live turtledove and burn it alive with its feathers, and take 1 ounce of frankincense, an equal amount of sandragon, and burn them to powder in an earthen pot. And have the woman use the powder in sauce, soup, and in drink. Also make a powder of 10 ounces each of burnt hartshorn and egg shells, and drink 2 drachms of this powder each treatment with the juice of plantain or [f. 203r] good moderate ale that is not strong, and her blood will be staunched. Also take 3 drachms each of Armenian bole, caraway seed, 1 drachm of ginger, 1 drachm of fine red coral; make a powder and give it to her and it will stop the flow of blood. A good medicine for a young girl's flux: take 2 drachms each of galingale, cinnamon, 3 drachms of red and white coral, 2 drachms each of sandragon and Armenian bole, 1 [drachm] each of gum arabic, of myrtle strained in a colander, half a drachm each of white and black plums, acacia, and licorice. Make a powder of these and give it to her with the juice of periwinkle, or make a powder of plantain, or of septfoil, roast bones, or mullein. Also take 1 drachm each of hypocistis, acacia,

---

* A plant that induces vomiting.

lapis ematites* ana ʒ i, make pouder & drynke it with jus of roses
or elles with rose water† or pouder of Athanasia, ʒ iii ydronke
with þe jus of sloue or elles a pissarie made of jus of sloue with
the newe pouder of athanasia & þat ycast into her prevy membre;
it staunchith it yf it be curable. Also, take bole fyne with þe jus off
planteyn & make a suppositorie with coton & yputt into þe prevy
membre; it helpith moche. Also, pouder of þe floure of rys, of
pomegarnadis, id est, balaustie with þe jus of sanguinarie‡ & so
ypissaried it is riȝt profitable. Or ellis menge turmentill, moleyne, roste bones, peruynka, virge pastoris, and sethe all these
in tanners wose þat is cleped amonge hem the fyrst becche &
whan they ben all ysoden, lete þe woman sytte theryn vp to þe
navell al so longe as sche may endure, for this is proved in Esex.
Also, pouder of corall þat is fyne & right rede & ydronke, hyt
staunchith all maner fluxes. Also maces and saffran togeders
staunchith it also. Item: take vitriole brent or vnbrent ʒ i & jus of
playntayn ʒ vii with þe stone of ematites ʒ i & caste it into prevy
membre [f. 203v] & it staunchith. Also, yf hir thenke that it
brennyth that comyth fro hyr at þe pryve membre, take than þe
muscillage of psillium & þe muscillage of þe sedes of quinces & of
þe gumme of draganti albi ana ʒ i, of womannes mylk ʒ vi, caste it
into þe prevy membre & this medecyn helith & staunchith all
blode þat comyth thorouȝ hote causes. Also, another preciouse
medecyne is this: Take saunders, the rede & þe white spodie,
sumak,§ mirtille ana ʒ ii, acacie ʒ iii, ypoquistydes ʒ iii, jus of
planteyne, jus of rede roses or the water of roses ana quartern iii,
barly mele as it sufficith; make a plaster of all these materiall fyrst
ypouderd and þat plaster schal be sumdel nesshe. Also, another
precius plaster is this: Whan þe blode is colerik, take the jus of
planteyne li. i, water of roses a quarteron, of vinegre ʒ sem., of
rede corall, of cacabri, of lapis amatiste, of bole armoniak, of
mirtill, of acornys cuppis, of olibani ana ʒ ii, of terre sigillate ʒ
sem.; all these ypouderd and hereof made two enplasters—oone
afore vnder þe navel & anoþer layd to behynde on þe raynes.
Also þe vtmest es bathe made of water þat alum de plume is
soden in for it is experte. And Avicen techith it in the 2ᵉ

*ematites: MS. ematiste (confused with amatist).
† his dotted for expunction before rose water.
‡ sanguinarie: MS. sanguarie.
§ sumak: MS. sumat.

the stone hematite,* make powder and drink it with the juice of roses or else with rose water or powder of Athanasia, 3 drachms drunk with the juice of sloe, or else have a pessary made of the juice of sloe with the fresh powder of Athanasia and cast into her privy member; it staunches if the condition is curable. Also, take fine Armenian bole with the juice of plantain, make a suppository with cotton, and put it into the privy member; it helps greatly. Also, powder of rice flower, of pomegranate, that is, the flower of wild pomegranate, with the juice of knotgrass made into a pessary is very helpful. Or else mix septfoil, mullein, roasted bones, periwinkle, shepherd's rod, and boil all these in tanners' juice that is called among them "the first run," and when they are all boiled let the woman sit in them up to her navel for as long as she can, for this has been tested in Essex.

Also, if fine bright red powder of coral is drunk, it staunches all manner of fluxes, as does mace and saffron. In addition take 1 ounce of vitriol burnt or unburnt, 7 ounces of the juice of plantain with 1 ounce of hematite, and cast it into the privy member, [f. 203v] and it will staunch. Also, if it seems to her that what comes from her at the privy member is burning, take then 1 ounce each of the oil from fleawort, quince seeds, and the gum of white tragacanth, 6 ounces of woman's milk, put it into the privy member, and this medicine heals and staunches all blood that comes through reasons of heat. Also, another valuable medicine is this: take 2 drachms each of sandalwood, the red and the white spode, sumac, myrtle, 3 drachms of acacia, 3 drachms of hypocistis, 3 measures each of the juice of plantain, juice of red roses or the water of roses, barley meal as necessary; make a plaster of all these materials first powdered, and the plaster should be somewhat soft. Also, another valuable plaster is this: when the blood is choleric, take 1 pound of the juice of plantain, a measure of water of roses, half a drachm of vinegar, 2 drachms each of red coral, gum, the stone amethyst,† Armenian bole, myrtle, acorn cups, olibanum, half a drachm of Lemnian earth; have all these powdered and made into two plasters—one in front under the navel and the other placed behind on the kidneys. For the greatest effect have a bath of water that some plume alum‡ has been boiled in, for it is a tested remedy. And Avicenna gives such instruction in the second

* Defined in *M.E.D.* as (a) a red iron ore; (b) bloodstone, heliotrope. See also Pliny, *N.H.*, XXXV, 144–48.
† Probably hematite is meant.
‡ See *M.E.D.* s.v. alum 3(c).

chapiter of bothe. Also vnderstonde yf the mater be right colrik, it is nede þat it be purged with medecyns þat purgen colre as thus: Take of mirabilanys citrini ʒ i, reubarbium ʒ *sem.*, puluerizentur & put her to diaprunis ʒ iii, electuarii de succo rosarum ʒ i, & medle hem togeder with the pulpe of cassia fistula as it sufficith to þe foresaid & drynke ʒ iii of whyt whaye þat borage was soden yn & whan this is done by thre or foure dayes than yeve her euer bytwene zucarum rosarum ʒ ii, poudre of Athanasia* newlich made [f. 204r] ʒ i with whyt zucarum cassatyne ʒ vi, ydrawen togeder drynke this with the jus aforesaid. And yf it staunche with none of these medecyns, do sette blode boxes on hir tetes with fyre & but these sufficen, God is medecyn and no man but he.

*The thyrde Chapiter is of þe Suffocacion of þe moder.*

Svffocacion of the moder is whan a womannes hert and her longes ben ythrust togeder by the moder that a woman semeth dede saue by her brethyng, & summe clepe it a cardiacle for it is a greuaunce of þe hert. For whan þer comyth a corupt smoke fro the moder and gothe up to þe hed otherwhile by þe riggebone into her hynder partie of þe hede, oþerwhile be þe brest into þe ferþer parte of þe heed, & for the brayne of woman is more myhgty than her herte, therfore that smoke may noȝt abyde in the hede but smytith downe into þe hert & grevith þe hert ful moche & makith the hert to closyn hym togeder more than he schuld do be kynde. And in this evell women fallen doune to þe grounde as þogh they hadde þe fallyng evel & liggen so in a swowe. And this akses endureth otherwhiles two dayes or thre. And this syknesse comyth of diuerse enchesons as of withholdyng of þe blode that they shuld ben purged of; other of sume corupt humours & venemous that ben in þe moder as men ben deliuered of sede that passith from her stones that ben by her yerde. And also men fallen into diuerse syknes for withholdyng of her sede within hem, riȝt so doeth women. But when women haue thys syknesse or than they fallen a downe, they felen moche ache & greuaunce from her navel dounward [f. 204v] & þei bowen her heed downe to her knees for greuaunce & withholden her wombe & clippen it harde togedre with her hondes and maken other men oþerwhiles to thryst her wombe togeder &

*Athanasia: MS. Anathasie.

chapter of both books. Also understand that if the matter is truly choleric it must be cleansed with medicines for purging choler thus: take 1 ounce of yellow plums, half an ounce of rhubarb, let them be crushed, add them to a medicament of 3 ounces of plums, 1 drachm of syrup of juice of roses, and mix them together with the pulp of cassia fistula as suffices, and drink 3 drachms of white whey that borage has been boiled in, and when this is done for three or four days, then give her every now and then 2 ounces of rose sugar, 1 ounce of newly made powder of Athanasia [f. 204r] with 6 ounces of white caffatin* sugar, put together and drunk with the beforementioned juice. And if none of these medicines staunch the blood, place blood boxes on her nipples with heat, and if these are of no use, only God can cure.

*The third chapter is concerned with the suffocation of the uterus.*

Suffocation of the uterus is when a woman's heart and lungs are thrust together by the uterus so that the woman seems dead except for her breathing, and some call it a heart attack because it is a malady of the heart. For when an evil fume comes from the uterus and goes up to the head, either by the backbone into the back part of the head or by the breast into the front part of the head, because a woman's brain is larger than her heart, the fume cannot stay in the head but strikes down into the heart, troubling it very much and making it tighten more than it naturally should. And in this sickness women fall to the ground as though they had the falling sickness and lie as though in a faint. And this pain lasts either two or three days. And this sickness is due to various reasons, such as the retaining of blood or of corrupt and venomous uterine humors that should be purged in the same way that men are purged of seed that comes from their testicles next to the penis. And just as men fall into various illnesses through retaining their seed within them, so do women. But when women have this sickness or when they fall down, they have great pain and discomfort from the navel downward, [f. 204v] and they bow their heads to their knees for distress, and hold their womb and clasp it hard together with their hands, and sometimes make other people thrust their womb together, and

* See *M.E.D.* s.v. caffatin.

88

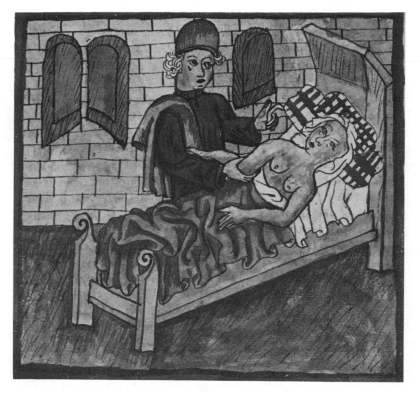

An unusual illustration from a fifteenth-century German manuscript of a physician taking the pulse at the brachial artery. The wrist was the usual place for pulse-taking, but texts also recommend the arm, foot, neck, or behind the ear.

they holden her teth togeder and sithen they falle downe to grounde as though they were dede; & oþerwhiles they beten þe erthe with her hondes and with her fete for þe gret greuaunce þat þei haue. And yf this greuaunce come of þe forsaid withholdyng of blode, men shall best knowen by þe pacientes tellyng, for she may best weten wheder she were purged of her blode as sche shuld be, other nay. But yf it is of corupt humours that ben in þe moder, that may be in two maners—as of hote humours oþer of cold. Yeff the humours be hote, she felith prykkyng and brennyng in þe depnesse of þe moder and þerof ben resolued hote smokes þat ben dispersid* thorough all þe body & makith

*dispersid: MS. disperlid.

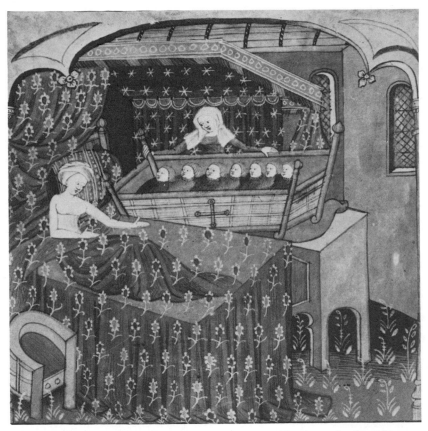

The mother of the Knight of the Swan is presented by the midwife with seven
newborn infants (MS. Roy 15, E VI, f. 273).

they hold their teeth together and afterward they fall down to
the ground as though they were dead; and sometimes they beat
the earth with their hands and feet because of the great pain
that they have. And if this sickness comes from the retention of
blood previously mentioned, one can best determine from what
the patient says, for she knows best whether she was purged of
her blood as she should be, or not. And if it is from corrupt
humors that are in the uterus, these may be of two kinds, either
hot or cold. If the humors be hot, she feels pricking and burning
in the cavity of the uterus, and loosening hot vapors that are
dispersed throughout the entire body, making

her to haue an vnkynde hete, in maner of a feuer, in hir body. But yf þe humour be colde than hath she moche heuynesse in þe depnesse of her moder & þerof is resolued a colde smoke that smytith vp to þe heued by þe riggebone & by þe stomak also. And she felith otherwhiles gret greuaunce aboute þe splene in the lyft syde. But if it be of corupt sede before, than þe greuaunce is withouten these foresaid tokens. But neuertheles, þe moder semyth replete of such moystnesse.

*Cura huius*: For to helpe women of this syknesse it is nedefull to porge þe moder of blode, yf it is in þe fyrst maner; or of þe corupt humours that ben in þe moder, yf it is in þe secunde maner other in the third maner. Nathelesse, yf it come in the third maner, it is profitable to haue company with man. But þus vnderstonde: in lawefull company-[f. 205r]yng, as with her housebandes and with none other; for in certayn it were better for a man other for a woman to haue þe grettest sekenesse of þe body the whiles þei leven than to ben helyd thorough a dede of lechery other ony other dede ayenst goddis hestys. And so by þat that is sayd before in þe Chapiter of withholdyng of blode, they mowe ben yholpen. Natheles, þat tyme that women hauen axes of this syknesse, they mowe receyve noo stronge medecyns to purgen hem but it be stronge women that ben of stronge complexion. And ther of, whan they ben in her axes, medle oyle de bay & oyle of roses togedre, of bothe yliche moche, and þerwith anoynt her armes & her hondes, her legges and her fete, & lete sette a blode glasse with fyre on her share withouten changyng. And lete her smelle stynkyng thinges that stynkyn horibely & foule as feltis ybrent oþer houndes heer, other gotes heer, other an horse bone ybrent & sithen yquenched, other herteshorne, oþer olde shone, oþer feþeres brent, oþer a wyke wet in oyle & ytende & sithen yquenched, oþer a wollen cloute, oþer a quyk cole so smokyng: lete her take that smoke, other take þe pouder of castory & galbanum resolued in vinegre & as moche of brymstone, parsilii, peusadanum, & put þerto a peny weight of petrolion, & lete cast all these on þe coles so þat þe smoke mowe come to her nose & in at her mouthe. Other take oyle comune *li.* ii, flours & leves of rosemary, nept, calamynt, pulegii, thym,* origany, isope, saueray, lorer leves, shavyng of cipresse ana ℥ & *sem.*, clowes & calami aromatici, ciperi, macis ana ℥ ii, myrra ℥ i, vini albi aromatici *li. sem.*, coquantur, id est, sethe hem tyl the wyne be

*thym: MS. thyn.

her have an unnatural heat, like a fever, in her body. But if the humor is cold, then she has much heaviness in the cavity of her uterus, loosening a cold vapor that strikes up to the head by the backbone and by the stomach also. And she feels at times great pain about the spleen on the left side. But if it comes from corrupt seed previously, then the pain is without these signs mentioned earlier. Even so, the uterus seems full of such moistness.

*The cure for this:*    To help women with this sickness one must purge the uterus of blood, if it is of the first kind; or of the corrupt humors that are in the uterus, if it is of the second or third kind. Nevertheless, if the ailment is of the third kind, it is helpful to have relations with a man. But understand what I have to say: the relations must be lawful, [f. 205r] such as with her husband and no other; for certainly it is better for man or woman to have the greatest physical illness while they live than to be healed through a deed of lechery or any other deed against God's commands. And so in this way, as I said before in the chapter on the retention of blood, they may be helped. Nevertheless, when women have an attack of this sickness, they may not receive any strong medicines to cleanse them unless they are strong women of strong constitution. And for this sickness, when they have an attack, mix bay oil* and oil of roses together, both an equal amount, and anoint their arms and hands, legs and feet with it, and have a heated bleeding glass put on the genitals without variation. And let the patient smell stinking things that are exceptionally odorous, such as burnt felt, dog's hair, goat's hair, or a horse's bone set alight and then extinguished, or hartshorn, old shoes, burnt feathers, a wick, moistened in oil, ignited and then extinguished, a woollen rag, or a live smoking coal. Let her smell that smoke, or take castory powder, galbanum dissolved in vinegar, an equal amount of brimstone, parsley, and hog's fennel, add to it a pennyweight of stone parsley, and throw all these on the coals so that the smoke may go into her nose and mouth. Alternatively, take 2 pounds of common oil, 1 drachms each of flowers and leaves of rosemary, catmint, calamint, fleawort, thyme, origanum, hyssop, savory, laurel leaves, a shaving of cypress, 2 drachms each of cloves and sweet calamus, galingale, mace, 1 drachm of myrrh, half a pound of white, sweet-smelling wine, and let them be cooked, that is to say, boil them until the wine is

*Made from the leaves of the laurel tree.

consumed & than clense it & cetera. And from [f. 205v] the navel
douneward to her prevy membre, lete anoynt here with wel
smellyng thinges as oynementes & oyles, & make her a fumigacion bynetheforth of wel smellyng thinges & swete, & drawe
þe mater fro the hert dounwarde. And suche thingis þat ben
good herefore ys gallia muscata, muske, xilocassie, aumber,
fraunkencense, storax liquida, calamus aromaticus, lignum
aloes, bawme, & suche thingis that haven a swote savour. And
also, in þe tyme of her axesse, lete bynde her legges & her thyes
togeder & frote wel þe soles of her fete with vyneger and salt.
And make her a fumigacion bynetheforthe of swete smellyng
thinges so þat þe smoke ne the savour come noȝt vp to her nose.
But lete her smellen azafetida & oþer stinkyng thingis, as I said
before. And make her to snesen with þe pouder of castory, of
peper, of euforbie, of piretrum ana ꝯ *sem.*, caste into her nose.
Other in tyme of her axes yef her triacle ȝ i and anoynt þe mouthe
of þe marice with wel smelling oynementes. A good fumigacion
to waken her in the tyme of her axes & speke: Take a peusadanum ȝ vii, of galbanum ȝ xii, of cost also moche, of peper xi
greynes and a litell baume tho that may be made into poudre;
poudre hem but resolue galbanum in vynegre & cast it on the
coles & let here hange her nose ouer þe smoke, & all these
medecyns schall be done in þe tyme of her axes whan she ys
fallen downe to grounde. But byfore & after thow myght gyfen
medecyns to make her to haue her purgacion as it is said before.
And yf þe humours be of colde that makith her to haue that
greuaunce, lete bathen her in a bath of hote herbes. And whan
she comyth outewardes of þe bath, yeve her a drawt [f. 206r] of
wyne that comyn and gynger ben soden yn. But yf it be of corupt
sede, lete her oftesithes be garsed bynethe the sparlyuer, bothe
behynde & before. And lete her blede also at þe veyne vnder the
ancle and atte her gret toon. And lete bray in a morter of brasse,
lovache, wormode, isop, & sote, and sithen sethe hem in water
and plastre it before, fro the mouthe of hyr stomak to hyr prevy
membre and also moche behynde on hyr bak, also on hyr sydes.
Sote also ysothen and yplasterd in þe same wise withowten ony
other þing helpith; other wormode by hymsylf helpith hem in
onys leggyng to hem though men do no more. Also take sal
gemme, sal nitri pouder and distempere hem with vynegre &
with salt water and wete a weke of coton therin & put it into hir
prevy membre & it wyll delyuer her of that corupt sede.

consumed, then strain it, etc. And from [f. 205v] the navel down to the privy member anoint her with fragrant things such as ointment and oils, and make a fumigation underneath of pleasant, sweet-smelling things and draw the matter down from the heart. And such things that are good for this are French muscat, musk, cassia wood, ambergris, frankincense, storax resin, sweet calamus, wood aloes, balm, and such things as have a fragrant smell. And also, at the time of her attack, bind her legs and thighs together and rub the soles of her feet well with vinegar and salt. And make her a fumigation underneath of sweet-smelling things so that neither the smoke nor the smell reaches her nose. But let her smell asafetida and other evil-smelling things as I said before. And make her sneeze with half a scruple each of the powder of castory, pepper, euphorbia, and pellitory put in her nose. Or, at the time of her attack, give her 1 drachm of medicinal syrup and anoint the mouth of the womb with sweet-smelling ointments. A good fumigation to make her wake up during her attack and speak: take 7 drachms of hog's fennel, 12 drachms of galbanum, an equal amount of costmary, 11 grains of pepper, and a little balm that may be made into powder; powder them but dissolve the galbanum in vinegar and throw it on the coals and let her hang her nose over the smoke, and all these medicines shall be given at the time of her attack when she is prostrate. But before and after you might give medicines to make her have her purgation, as said before.

And if cold humors cause her complaint, let her bathe in a bath of hot herbs. And when she comes out of the bath, give her a draft [f. 206r] of wine that cumin and ginger are boiled in. But if her sickness is the result of corrupt seed, let her often be lanced under the calf, both behind and in front. And let her bleed also at the vein under the ankle and at her big toes. And have lovage, wormwood, hyssop, and soot ground together in a brass mortar, and afterward boil them in water and plaster the liquid in front, from the mouth of her stomach to her privy member, and also a considerable amount behind on her back as well as on her sides. Soot boiled and plastered in the same way without anything else is helpful; or wormwood by itself helps in a single application, though one do no more. Also take rock salt, saltpeter, and blend with vinegar and salt water and wet a wick of cotton in them, put it in her privy member, and it will free her from that bad seed.

94

And beth they war of metes* that encresith sede bothe in a man &
in a woman, & suche metis ben yelkis of eyren and fressh flessh
& nameliche of swyne, of cokkes, of sparewys, partryches,
quayles and brayne of a bore & þe stones of bestes, as of bores, of
boles, of wolues principalliche, and þe mary & the fatnesse and
þe brayne of bestes; pyries, dates, almaundes, fygges, nuttes,
pastinakes, rapys fryed with honye & oyle of benen & pesyn &
stronge, swete wyne & saturnous; and good wyne þat is myghty
& swete, bothe whit & rede, & mete also & moche reste & slepe &
likyng in bathes. Also so that they dwelle not longe in the bath
but lete vsen suche thingis that wastith† & consumyth seed as
fastyng & wakyng, isop & rue & comyn that thoroughe her hete
consumen þe seed. And other thingis menusith the seed as colde
herbes [f. 206v] as agnus castus, water lilies, & suche other. Also
yf the mydwyf wete her handes in oyle of puliol & in oile
muschiling ana ʒ iii medled togeders and thanne anoynte þe
orifice of her pryve membre, it shulde make tykelyng in þe
marice. And for she wil come douneward with swete smellyng
thynges, now to take oyle muschilyng þou schalt doon thus:
Take two galons and half of good mete oyle that is riʒt swete, and
put þerto a li. of puliole riall, of rosemaryn, of cost, of camomille,
lauendre, of baume, of woderove, of isope, saturei, and shavyng
of cipresse ana li. sem., of calamynt, of fethrefew, of fenell, of
wormode, of sauge, of rue, of origanum, of sothernewode, of
mugwede of S. Johannes, id est, herbe John worte ana ʒ xii;
wasshe hem fyrst in water & sethe hem in maluesyn & grynde
hem & put hem into þe oile aforesaid & put therto of þat wyne a
quart and so lete þe herbes rote in þe oile with þat maluesyn a ix
dayes or ellis more yf þou myghtyst. Than anone do sethe all
these in a double glasse ouer the fyre & lete hem sethe right wel
till they haue nyʒe consumed; than clense it thorouʒ a fayre
newe canvasse þat is wyde threded & whan this is clensed, make
this pouder. R_x: lignum aloes, maces, carpobalsami, xilobalsami,
calami aromatici, nardi, ciperi, masticis, croci, garriofoli, mirre,
galange, rasure cipressi ana ʒ ii, calamini aromatici, storacis,
calamynte ana ʒ ii & sem., musci boni, camphore ʒ vi, ambre Ə ii;
grynde thy campher & thy muske & than medle hem with oyle ʒ
ii, but all þe tother saue these thre, id est, campher & muske &
storax shal noʒt be put into oyle tyl þe spices be

*MS. margin: Metes to encre sperme.
† MS. margin: To waste sperme.

And one should guard against foods that increase the seed in both a man and a woman, and such foods are yolks of egg, fresh meat, especially of swine, cocks, sparrows, partridges, quails, boar's brain, and the testicles of animals, such as boars, bulls, and wolves principally, and the marrow and fat and brain of animals; pears, dates, almonds, figs, nuts, parsnip, turnip fried with honey and oil of beans and peas; strong, sweet, full-bodied wine, good wine that is strong and sweet, both white and red; food, much rest and sleep, and fondness for baths. Also, they should not stay in the bath long but use such things as exhaust and destroy the seed, such as fasting and keeping awake, hyssop, rue and cumin, which through their heat destroy the seed. And other things reduce the seed, such as cold herbs [f. 206v] like St.-John's-wort, water lilies, and similar things. Also, if the midwife wets her hands in 3 drachms each of oil of wild thyme and oil of musk mixed together, and then anoints the orifice of the privy member, an itching in the womb should result. And so that the matter may be brought down with sweet-smelling things, take the oil of musk and do thus: take 2½ gallons of good, suitable oil that is very sweet and add to it 1 pound of pennyroyal, half a pound each of rosemary, costmary, camomile, lavender, balm, woodruff, hyssop, savory, shaving of cypress, 12 drachms each of calamint, feverfew, fennel, wormwood, sage, rue, origanum, southernwood, mugwort of St.-John's, that is, the herb Johnwort; wash them first in water, then boil in malmsey, grind them up, put them in the previously mentioned oil, add to the mixture a quart of wine, and let the herbs rot in the oil with the malmsey for nine days or more if you can. Then shortly boil all these ingredients in a double glass over the fire and let them boil right down until they are almost nothing; then pass them through a good, new, wide-meshed canvas to clean them, and when they are strained make this powder: take 2 ounces each of wood aloes, mace, carpobalsam,* balsam wood, aromatic calamus, spikenard, galingale, mastic, saffron, cloves, myrrh, galingale, shaving of cypress, 2½ drachms each of aromatic calamus, gum, and calamint, good musk, 6 drachms of camphor, 2 scruples of ambergris; grind your camphor and musk, and then mix them with 2 drachms of oil, all the rest except these three, that is, camphor, musk, and gum shall not be put in the oil until the spices are

* Fruit of one kind of balsam tree.

grounden & soden in [f. 207r] that oyle in a glasen vessell, & whan it is nygh cold, putte in the storax; but whan it is riȝt cold, putte in þe camphre & muske & þe aumbre & do it vp for it is neuer the wors though it stonde on þe leys.* For this oyle is good for all maner of syknesse þat comyn, namely of colde & specially for the suffocacion of þe marice. Yf it be anoynted þerwith withinforth or els coton ywet theryn & vnder putt, it provokith þe marice & comfortith it. Also þis oyle is for the coldnesse of þe stomak yf it be anoynted þerwith and also for þe feuers tercian oþer quartain oþer cotidian þat comyn thorough fleume naturall, yf þe pacient be anoynted with this oyle afore þe houre of his axes. Anoynt wel his ryggebones; it for-nemyth the quakyng of þe feuers & moche more; if þe pacient drynk þerof ʒ i with good fyne maluesyn ʒ iiii a two houres afore his axes, it shal make þat his axes shall nouȝt come. This oyle is good ayen colde paralises, colde rewmes, yef the nape† of þe nek be anoynted therwith. Also, this oyle doth away all maner of aches that comyn thorough colde yf they be anoynted therwith. Also for all maner of colde gowtes it is good to anoynt therwith, and colde ydropisies, and all suche other. Also þe rote of yres vnder put into þe marice oþer subfumygid with yres makith her to lessen her chylde, for yres rotes ben hote & drye & haue vertu to opyne & to hete & to consume & waste. For whan the woman is feble & þe chyld may noȝt comyn out, than it is better that þe chylde be slayne than the moder of þe child also dye. And also it bringeth forth þe dede chyld mervelously & þe secundine & menstrua with hit. Sub-fumigate or [f. 207v] ellis take *li. sem.* of his‡ rotes and of savyne ʒ *sem.*, & sethe hem in whyt wyne & do her to pouder of paulini ʒ i, hony ʒ i, of that decoction quartern i, bolys galle ʒ i, & make a pissarie & yeve troscisci de murra ʒ ii with this decoction. Rₓ: Ameos, woderove, parcely sede, baume, carui, anete, iris, mugwede, ana ʒ i, whyt wyne *li.* iii.
Sethe hem; than grynde saueray, isop, woderoue, diptayne ana ʒ i, tempre it vp with ʒ iiii of the decoction, & cetera.

*leys: MS. seys.
† nape: MS. nede. Sloane 249, f. 190, also has nede. Nape is written above in a different hand.
‡ his: scribal error for iris.

mixed and boiled in [f. 207r] that oil in a glazed vessel, and when the decoction is nearly cold, put in the gum; and when it is very cold, put in the camphor, musk, and ambergris, and close it up, for it is never the worse, even though it stands in the lees. For this oil is good for all kinds of sickness that occur, especially for cold and for the suffocation of the womb. If it is used for anointing inside, or if cotton moistened with it is applied, it stimulates the womb and comforts it. Also, this oil can be used for anointing in cases of coldness of the stomach and also for tertian, quartan, and quotidian fevers that are a result of natural phlegm, provided that the patient is anointed with this oil one hour before the time of his attack. Oil the backbone well; it takes away the shivering due to the ague and much more; if the patient drinks 1 ounce of it with 4 ounces of good, fine malmsey two hours before his attack, it will cause his attack to come to nothing. This oil is good for cold paralysis, catarrhal colds, if the nape of the neck is oiled with it. Also, this oil does away with all kinds of aches that come as a result of a cold, if the patients are oiled with it. It is also good for all kinds of cold gouts, cold dropsies, and similar things. Also, the root of iris put into the womb or fumigated underneath makes a woman lose her child, for iris roots are hot and dry and have the virtue of opening, heating, consuming, and wasting. For when the woman is feeble and the child cannot come out, then it is better that the child be killed than the mother of the child also die. And also the medicament brings out the dead child marvellously, and the secundine, and menstrual fluid. Subfumigate or [f. 207v] else take half a pound of iris roots and half an ounce of savin, boil them in white wine, and add to half an ounce of powder of ground ivy, 1 ounce of honey; with 1 measure of the boiled proceeds, take 1 drachm of bull's gall, and make a pessary, and give a pill of 2 drachms of myrrh with this liquid. Take 1 ounce each of bishop's-weed, woodruff, parsley seed, balm, caraway, dill, iris, artemisia, and 3 pounds of white wine.

Boil them; then chop up 1 ounce of savory, hyssop, woodruff, and dittany in equal amounts, dilute with 4 drachms of the liquid, etc.

*The 4 Chapeter is of the precipitacion of the moder.*

The precipitacion of þe moder is another syknesse whan þe moder fallith fro hir kyndely place into anoþer place & þat may be in two maners: oþer asyde other ellis douneward. Yf it fallith asyde men may it knowe by the greuaunce of þe side; douneward it may fallen in two maners: other all owte of þe wombe or els nouȝt fully oute. Yef hit falle not fulliche oute, they felen moche greuaunce aboue þe share & aboute þe raynes. And yf it goth all aboute, þe woman may sene þat hersylf. This syknesse comyth ofte of withholdyng of blode þat women shuld haue ben ypurged of; or els of corupt humours that ben in þe moder þat makith hir to fallen a downe or aside; other þe moder fallyth a downe oute att þe wombe for þe paralisi þat þe moder hath caught thorough colde in longe sitting on cold stones or suche oþer wey; other thorough longe abydyng in a colde bath; other for moche drynkyng of cold water. And whan þe moder hath this paralisi, she fallith downe out at þe wombe withouten greuaunce oþer ache; otherwhiles þe moder fallith oute for greuaunce þat a woman hathe in [f. 208r] beryng of child. And yf this greuaunce come of withholdyng of hir blode oþer of corupt humours that ben in þe moder that thristeth her oute of hyre place wheder þat they be hote or colde, þou myht knowe hit by þe tokenes that weren ytolde in the next chapeter. And than the syknesse is helyd yf þe moder be purged of þe blode þat is withholden oþer of þe corupt humours that ben within hyr as hit was tolde before. But yf it come of þe paralisi of þe moder, lete her vsen the oximelle þat was ytolde bifore. And afterward gyve here theodoricon empiricon. Afterward, on þe third day, make her a stuphe of calamynt, of origanum, of lauendre, of sauge, of kersis, of primeros, of confery, & of rue. And whan she comyth fro þe stuphe, yeve her triacle with wyne that sauge is soden yn. And þe next daye after, lete her bleden at þe veyne vnder þe ancle. And make her an oynement of clotes & oyle of nottys & wey yfryed togeder and ywrongen thorough a clothe, & sithen caste þeron pouder of encense & mastik & with this anoynt her from þe navell douneward bothe behynde & before. *Item*: þe jus of ipie minoris dronken with wyne clarre twyes a day wyl drawen vp þe marice; other els medle the jus of clotes & agrippa togeders ouer the fyre & þerwith anoynt her bothe before & behynde—& before from þe navel dounwardes—& ther aboue

*The fourth chapter is concerned with the precipitation of the uterus.*

The precipitation of the uterus is another sickness that occurs when the uterus falls from its natural place to another place, and it can be in two ways: either sideways or downward. If the womb falls sideways, one can tell by the pain in the side; it falls downward in two ways: it either falls right out or not fully out. If it does not fall fully out, women feel great pain about the genitals and the kidneys. If it goes all the way, the woman can see it for herself. This illness is often due to the retention of the blood that women should lose; or to evil humors that are in the uterus, which make it fall down or sideways; or the uterus falls out because of paralysis caught through cold, through sitting for a long time on cold stones or in some such way, or through staying too long in a cold bath or drinking too much cold water. And when the uterus has this paralysis, it falls out at the opening without pain or discomfort; or the uterus falls out because of the illness that a woman has in [f. 208r] bearing a child. And if this illness is due to the retention of blood or corrupt humors that are in the uterus and cause distortion whether they are hot or cold, you can know by the signs described in the adjoining chapter. And then the sickness is cured if the uterus is purged of the blood that is retained or the corrupt humors that are inside, as was described before. But if the ailment is a result of paralysis of the uterus, let the patient use oxymel, which was mentioned before. And afterward give her theodoricon empiricon, and on the third day make her a bath of calamint, origanum, lavender, sage, cresses, primrose, comfrey, and rue. And when she comes from the bath, give her a sovereign remedy with wine that sage is boiled in. And the following day bleed the vein under the ankle. And make her an ointment of burdock, oil of nuts, and whey fried together and rung through a cloth, and afterward throw on it incense powder and mastic, and with this mixture anoint her from the navel downward both in front and behind. Also, the juice of chickweed drunk in clary twice a day will draw up the womb; or else mix the juice of burdocks and agrippa* together over the fire and anoint her with the mixture both behind and in front, and in front from the navel downward, and

* A herb used for unguents.

ley þe wolle of a shepe þat is yshore vnwasshen; other anoynt her aboue þe schare & aboute þe raynes with hote hony & theron strewe þe pouder of mastyk & of encense & of hertys hornys ybrent & of colophonie, other [f. 208v] of picche & þe pouder of kerseed, and sithen hile her with askes on that anoyntyng bothe before & behynd. And þe same medecynes ben gode yf it come out for cause of colde humours that ben within the modere. But yf it come of hote humours, gyve her a lectuarie de succo rosarum. And after that, make her a stuphe of cold herbes and afterward lete her bleden atte þe veyne vnder þe ancle and anoynt her with cold oynementis & with colde oyles; other take as moche of hony as of oyle & caste pouder of comyn to hem & sethe hem togeder. And afterward, wete þerin wolle of a shepe that is not wasshen oþer a blake felt & ley it from þe navel douneward & sume what aboue. But yf þe moder falle oute of the wombe bynetheforthe atte priue membre yf yt be whan she hathe borne child, lete þe mydwyf put it in ayen with her honde. But anoynte she her honde first with oile & sithen make her a fumygacion bynetheforth of maythes other of drieȝe ox dirt cast on þe coles. And lete hir smelle wel sauered thinges; other yf þe moder wil not liȝtly ben put in ayenward, sethe coste & wormode & mugwede in water, & do þe woman in þat water þe whiles it is warme vp to þe tetes & lete hyr sitte þerin a good while. Afterward, whan she is comyn oute of þe water, lete put þe moder softelich in ayen & heve hir feet & hir leggis higher than hyr heued, liggyng so ix houres of þe day, þat þe moder may go into here kyndely place. And whan þe moder is in, take þe pouder of these thingis, of gallee, muste, of nuttimiges, of spikenard, of clowes, & pouder hem alle in fere & tempre þat pouder with [f. 209r] oile of puliole* & do that into a small lynnen bagge of small & of softe clothe & make it of þe shappe of an evelonge balle after þe schappe of an eye, & put þat balle into þe prevy membre & let þe moder þat she falle not oute ayeneward, & bynde it with a sweþeles aboute her reynes þat it falle noght oute ayen. But or þou bynde þat swetheles, make a plaster aboute her reynes of þe pouder of kerseseed & of baye, of þe lorer, of comyn, & of wyld myntes; hatte in a vessell ouer þe fyre & sithen medled with hony & lete hym ligge thus ix dayes & in the mene tyme lete hir dieten hir with metes & with drinkes that she haue noon nede to goon oftesithes to þe prevy chambre ne to maken water;

*puliole: MS. piliole.

put on it the wool of a sheep that is shorn unwashed; or anoint her above the genitals and about the kidneys with warm honey, and strew on powder of mastic, incense, burnt hartshorn, colophony, or [f. 208v] pitch, and the powder of cress seed, and afterward cover her with ashes on the place anointed, both in front and behind. And the same medicines are effective for cold humors that are in the uterus. If the sickness is due to hot humors, give her a syrup of rose juice. And after that, make her a bath of cold herbs and then let her bleed at the vein under the ankle and anoint her with cold ointments and oils; or take as much honey as oil and throw cumin powder on them and boil them together. And then wet unwashed sheep's wool or black felt and put it on from the navel downward, and to a certain extent above. But if the uterus fall out underneath at the privy member after childbirth, let the midwife put it in again with her hand. But let her anoint her hand first with oil and afterward make a fumigation underneath of stinking camomile or of dry ox dirt thrown on the coals. And let her smell fragrant things; or if the uterus cannot easily be put in again, boil costmary, wormwood, and artemisia in water and place the woman in the water while it is warm up to her nipples and let her sit in it for a good time. Afterward, when she has come out of the water, put the uterus gently in again and raise her feet and legs higher than her head lying thus nine hours of the day, so that the uterus may go into its natural place. And when the uterus is in, take the powder of these things, gall, must, nutmegs, spikenard, cloves, powder them all together, mix the powder with [f. 209r] oil of wild thyme, place in a small linen bag of fine, soft cloth, make it the shape of an elongated ball similar in shape to an egg, and put that ball in the privy member to prevent the uterus from falling out again, and bind the uterus with a bandage about her loins, so that it does not fall out again. But before you use the bandage, make a plaster about her loins of the powder of cress seed, bay, laurel, cumin, and wild mint; put in a vessel over the fire and afterward mix with honey and let it remain thus nine days, and in the meantime let her eat and drink such things that will not require her to go often to the privy, nor to urinate.

otherwhiles sume women haue so gret penaunce in beryng of a childe that þe skynne þat is bitwen the two prevy membres brekith atwo & all is an hole, & so þe moder fallith out þeratte & wexith hard. To helpe women of þis mischief, fyrst sethe butter & wyne togedre halfe an houre; and all warme lete legge it to þe moder & softely handel þe moder & softely tawen it with þat wyne a good whiles to make þe moder nesshe, & sithen putte it in softely ayen & sowe togeder þat pece that is tobroken with a silken threde with a quarell nedell in thre places or in foure, and sithen do picche on a softe lynnen clothe & leye it to þe prevy membre & þe stynche of þat pitche shal make hyr to drawen hir inward to hir owne place. Afterward, make pouder of þe rote of comfery & of canell & strawe that in þe sore forto it be hole. And lete hir liggen, as I sayde [f. 209v] rather, a sevyne dayes or a nyne and lete her eten and drynken in þat while but litell and kepe hem well from colde & fro metes and drynkes that myght maken her eny coghe. And for to kepe women from this myschef in þat tyme that they traveyllen of childe, lete make a rounde thyng of þe shappe of an eye of small lynnen clothe, and putte it in her fundement and euerich tyme of chylde and eueryche suche tyme, lete thrust þat balle in her fundement & þat shal sauen þe skyn hole from brekyng. But in þe precipitacion of þe moder sixe thinges ben nedefull: the first is ventusyng and that in thre stedes. The fyrste is a litell vnder þe navel, but Lilie seyth þat it shuld be done on the tetes and oon on eyther halfe þe sydes of þe woman, and that is done for the marice shuld arise vp into her owne stede ayen. The seconde thyng is subfumigacion and þat is with an instrument that is cleped Embotum & it is made thus: take a litell erthyn potte þe while the woman shall siten on a sege with an hole on þat sege, and in þat litell potte shullen fyry coles ben putte þerin & that is shytte aboute with clothes, but embotum, id est, a litell pipe shall be on þe ouer ende off þat potte & þe women shall nyme þe smoke by þat instrument so that þe instrument shall entre into þat prevy membre of þe woman, & þe poudre shall be putt into þe coles vnder þe woman. Take tormentill, acacie, þe rotys of bistorte, serepium ana ʒ iii, persidie, balaustie ana ʒ ii & *sem.*, galange, nucis sipressi, foliorum galbani, mirte ana ʒ v, make poudre. Cause is why this pouder is made of stynking spyces and stiptyk; for stynke makith þe marice [f. 210r] to arise into hir place; but bewarre þat none of þat stynche come to þe womannes nose. But she schal holde sume thyng þat is of swete smell atte here nose & this shall be done the

Sometimes women have such difficulty in bearing a child that the skin between the two privy members breaks apart and is just a hole, and so the uterus falls out there and grows hard. To help women in this trouble, first boil butter and wine together for half an hour; and when the liquid is all warm put it in the uterus, handling the uterus kindly and treating it tenderly with that wine for a good while to soften the uterus, and afterward put it gently in again and sew together the piece that is broken with a silk thread and square needle in three or four places, and then put pitch on a soft linen cloth and apply to the privy member, and the stench of the pitch will make the womb draw inward to its place. Afterward, make a powder of the root of comfrey and cinnamon and straw and put it on that sore until it be whole. And let her lie, as I said [f. 209v] earlier, seven or nine days and drink and eat little during that time and keep well away from cold and from food and drink that might make her cough at all. And to prevent this trouble when women are in childbirth, make a round thing, the shape of an egg, from fine linen cloth and put it in her anus and with every pang of the child and indeed with every childbirth, thrust the ball into her anus, and that will keep the skin completely from breaking.

But in the precipitation of the uterus, six things are necessary: first is cupping, and that in three places. The first place is a little under the navel, but Lilie says that the cupping should be done on the nipples and one on each side, and that is done in order that the womb may rise up into its own place again. Second thing is subfumigation, and that is done with an instrument called a syringe, and it is made thus: take a little earthen pot while the woman sits on a bench with a hole in it, and in that little pot put fiery coals and cover with cloths, and the syringe, that is, a little pipe, should be at the upper end of the pot, and the woman takes the smoke through that instrument so that the instrument goes into her privy member, and the powder shall be put in the coals under her. Take 3 drachms each of septfoil, acacia, the roots of shakeweed, orchis, 2 drachms each of parsley, pomegranate flowers, 5 drachms each of galingale, seed of the cypress, leaves of galbanum, myrtle, and make powder. The reason that this powder is made of evil-smelling spices and styptic is that the stench makes the womb [f. 210r] rise into its place; but see that none of the stench reaches the woman's nose. She should hold to her nose something that has a sweet smell, and this should be done

whiles þat þe ventosing boistes ben on þe wombe; and Auicen seith 3°: also a bath is good in these nedes. Take rede rose leves ʒ ii, mirte, þe rotes of moleyn ana *m*. ii, turmentille, rotis of bistorte,* antere, mastik, olibani ana ʒ iiii, asefetide ʒ iiii, mugwede drie, lauendre drie ana ʒ ii, bete all these in a morter and putte hem in a poket and sethe it in a litel raspaise. And this bagge, be it dreynt in þe bath with smethis water and this is good for it is made of stinkyng & stiptik thinges. Also 4°, it askith to haue an oynement to anoynt with þe mouthe of þe prevites & þe parties of her reynes and is this: Take olibanum, mirtill, oile of lilie, oile of mastik ana ʒ vi, asefetide, rotis of bistorte, turmentill ana ʒ iii, cere ʒ iii. The 5° also is suppositorie made thus: R$_x$: asefetide ʒ i, masticis, olibani, sedis of mirtill, galange, nucis cipressi ana ʒ i, make pouder and tempre it vp with oyle of mirtill & make a suppositorie. The 6° is that a plastre be ordeyned on þe prevy membre lest þe marice falle ayen; and þat plastre shal be quantite of a pawme of þe honde & may be made thus: Take mastik ʒ iiii, olibani ʒ *sem*., nucis sipressi, gallarum, mirtill ana ʒ i, persidie, balaustie ana *sem*., turbenti ʒ i; make pouder† of all tho that may be pouderd and tempre it vp with oile of roses & make herof an emplaster & in brede of vi fyngerniele, in lengthe of viii or x fyngerniele. And make that plastre thyn. Also make the woman to spewe moche for it is one of [f. 210v] the best that may be don þerto. Also nym hede that all maner stinking thinges in this cause schull ben putte benetheforthe; and all maner of swete smelling thynges to þe nose in this cause.

*The 5 Chapiter ys of wynde of the moder.*

Moche wynde ther is also in þe moder þat grevith women ful moche and that comyth oþerwhile fro withouʒt, oþerwhile fro withyn that makith þe moder to ake & to swelle. And the tokens of suche wynde ben swelling and moche hurlyng and noyse withinforthe & gnawyng of þe wynde within þe moder. And for this siknesse, hem is good to vsen electuaries that wil consume and destroie wyndes. And such electuaries ben diaciminum, dianisum, diaspermaton; and oþer þinges of liʒt cost wyl destroye suche wyndes as comyn, anete, anisi, fenel sede, carui, apii, loueache, kersede, paritorie bothe emplasterd withouten &

*bistorte: MS. historte.
† pouder: MS. poouder.

during the time that the cupping boxes are on the womb; and Avicenna says thirdly: likewise, a bath is good in these necessities. Take 2 drachms of red rose leaves, myrtle, 2 handfuls of mullein root, 4 ounces of septfoil, roots of shakeweed, rose pollen, mastic, olibanum, 4 drachms of asafetida, 2 drachms each of dry artemisia, dry lavender, pound all these in a mortar, and put them in a bag, and boil them in a little raspberry wine. And if this bag is immersed in the bath with blacksmith's water, it is good, because it is made of evil-smelling and styptic things. Fourthly, an ointment is necessary to anoint the mouth of the privities and the parts of the kidneys, and it is this: take 6 drachms each of olibanum, myrtle, oil of lily, and oil of mastic, 3 drachms each of asafetida, roots of shakeweed, septfoil, and wax. Fifthly, a suppository is made thus: take 1 drachm each of asafetida, mastic, olibanum, myrtle seeds, galingale, and cypress seed; make a powder, dilute with oil of myrtle, and make a suppository. Sixthly, a plaster should be put on the privy member in order to prevent the womb from falling again; and that plaster should be the size of the palm of the hand and can be made thus: take 4 ounces of mastic, half an ounce of olibanum, 1 drachm each of seeds of cypress, oak apples, and myrtle, half [a drachm] each of parsley and wild pomegranate, 1 drachm of terebinth resin; make a powder of all those that can be powdered, dilute with oil of roses, and make a plaster six fingernails in breadth and eight or ten fingernails in length. And make that plaster thin. Also make the woman vomit a lot, for it is one of [f. 210v] the best things for it. Also, see that all kinds of evil-smelling things are put underneath for this condition; and all kinds of sweet-smelling things applied to the nose.

*The fifth chapter is concerned with wind in the uterus.*

There is also much wind in the uterus that distresses women exceedingly, and it comes sometimes from without, sometimes from within when it causes the uterus to ache and swell. And the signs of such wind are swelling, much movement and noise inside, and griping of the wind within the uterus. And for this sickness it is good for them to use electuaries that will consume and destroy winds. And such electuaries are a drug made from cumin, an electuary made from anise, and a drug made from seeds, and other things of little expense will destroy wind, such as cumin, dill, anise, fennel seed, caraway, wild celery, lovage, cress seed, pellitory put on in a plaster both outside and

withyn. Also in maner of medecyn a plaster made of comyn & of
sote ysoden in water; wasshe her wombe þerwith wel doune to
þe prevy membre; & also layde to þe wombe hote is riȝt profitable
ayenst þe wynde ouerall. Oþer, let her bathe her in water where
hokkis & paritorie ben soden in & wasshe wel her wombe with
the herbes. And sche comyth oute of þe bathe, let her haue a
plastre of paritorie al warme as she may suffre & ley it to her bely.
Other let sethe saveyn & rapes in water, & with þat water wasshe
her wombe wel doune to þe prevy membre. And this also is
profitable. Other medecyns þer beith þat ben good for stiches
and for wyndes in a mannes body & in his guttes ben good for
this syknesse, as a [f. 211r] plaster made of colver dirt soden in
wyne oþer the wyne ydronke. Other take hote shepes dirt and
stampe it in a morter with gotes mylk and afterward lete caste
þerto a litell quantite of picche; & fyre hem wel togeder and
sithen plastre it vp in a pece of leder & ley it warme to þe wombe;
oþer take þe erthe þat is tofore a bestes manger that is to-trede
with þe bestis fete & by-perysshed and hete þat erth wel ayenst
þe fyre and ley it there as þe greuaunce is, and make her abstene
her fro metes þat be wyndy as ben pesen & benes & fecches &
rawe frutes & rawe herbes. Also for þe wynde in þe moder: take
pouder of comyn, of anete, of galangale, of zeduale, of carui ana
ʒ iii, spikenard, canell, cokell ana ʒ i, castory ʒ sem., hony ʒ iii,
terbenti ʒ i; make a suppositorie of alle these thingis aforesaid &
putt it into þe prevy membre & it shal consume all maner wyndes
& foule retencions of þe marice and alle stenches. Also leves of
nettell* ygrounde & vnder putt anone it makith falleng women to
risen hole. Also rue grounde & sode with grece of hennes or off
ganders and hote layde before & behynde anone it helith. Also
netle seed with wyne dronke fordoth swelling and wynde. Also
doth xv graynes of pionys soden in wyne & dronke fordothe
suffocacion of þe moder & helpith that sorowe. Also derstes of
oyle yhette & with oyle put in it fordothe all þe swellyng of þe
marice. Item: so doth terbentyn, so dothe þe fomentacion origani
[yclensed]† & pressaried & so doth savyne & so don bitter
almaundes yclensed & grounde & putte yn bringeth forthe all
inneter‡ & all þe corupt humours of þe body. And so doth
aristologia with hony [f. 211v] and put in; also mirre

*MS. of, after nettell, dotted for expunction.
† yclensed supplied from next line.
‡ inneter: MS. inster.

inside. Also by way of remedy, have a solution made of cumin and soot boiled in water; wash her stomach with it right down to the privy member; and placed hot to the stomach, the medicament is very helpful against wind altogether. Or have the patient bathe in water in which mallow and pellitory are boiled, and wash her vulva well with the herbs. And when she comes out of the bath, let her have a plaster of pellitory as hot as she can bear, and place it on her belly. Alternatively, boil savin and turnips in water, and with that water wash her stomach down well to the privy member. And this is also helpful. Other medicines that are good for stitches and for winds in a man's body and in his guts are good for this sickness, such as [f. 211r] plaster made from the droppings of doves boiled in wine, or one may drink the wine. Another recipe is to take hot sheep's dung, mash it in a mortar with goat's milk, and then add a small quantity of pitch; burn them well together and afterward put them in the form of a plaster in a piece of leather and place it warm on the stomach. Or take the earth that is in front of a beast's manager that has been trodden on by the animal's feet and spoiled, heat that earth well upon the fire, lay it where the trouble is, and make her abstain from foods that are windy, such as peas, beans, vetches, raw fruits, and raw herbs. Also, for wind in the uterus: take 3 drachms each of powder of cumin, dill, galingale, setwall, and caraway, 1 drachm each of spikenard, cinnamon, and cockle, half a drachm of castory, 3 ounces of honey, 1 ounce of terebinth resin; make a suppository of all these things mentioned and put it into the privy member, and it will destroy all kinds of winds, foul retentions of the womb, and all evil smells. Also, nettle leaves ground and put underneath immediately cure afflicted women. Also, rue ground and boiled in the fat of hens or ganders and placed hot in front and behind immediately cures. Also, nettle seed drunk with wine destroys swelling and wind. Also, 15 grains of peonies boiled in wine and drunk destroy suffocation of the uterus and help that grievance. Also, dregs of oil heated and oil added destroy all the swelling of the womb. Again, so do terebinth resin, fomentation of origanum, purified and pressed,* and so do savin, bitter almonds cleaned, ground, and applied, bring out all that is inside and all the evil humors of the body. And so does birthwort with honey [f. 211v] put inside; also, myrrh

---

* From late Latin *pressorium*: a press for wine.

ydronke with the [jus] of arithimisie doth marvelous; so doth saturei putt yn bryngith forth dede childe.

*Off to moche Flux.* Make a suppositorie of gos oþer* gotes donge with þe jus of sanguinarie† and put vnder, staunchith all blody flux. So doth a bath of planteyn, of þe myddel ryndes of an oke, virge pastoris, sanguinarie‡ & suche other empericon§ ydronke, staunchith fluxe of þe wombe.

For the woo after þe birthe: take ʒelkes of eyren soden in water & gronde cera & oleo & succo arthimisie & cimino pouderd, and make an emplastre byfore & behynde & anone the penaunce shal sese. Also, yf she haue feuers, take oynonnes soden in water and grounde with þe yelkis of eyren soden in water with oile & poudre of comyn, and make an emplastre.**

Ydropisie of þe moder comyth otherwhiles of withholdyng of blode þat a woman shuld be purged of, & than she may noʒt ben heled but she be purged of þat blode; otherwhiles it comyth of wynde & of fleumatyk humours þat ben in þe moder and than a woman swellith with this ydropesie as þoughe sche were with childe. And þer ben many diuerse tokens to knowe oone from another;†† for this swelling comyth sodenly, the oþer ydropisies do not so. This swelling comyth oþerwhiles & oþerwhiles vanyshith away but þe toþer abidith alwey to a woman be de-liuered of a child; this walkith fro place to place; þe oþer doth noʒt so. Also this hath vncertayn mevinges but þe toþer mevith certanliche & atte þe certayne tymes bothe in þe day & also in þe nyght. But þe [f. 212r] ydropesie of þe moder, the mevyng & þe steryng, is oftesithes by nyght and selden be day. Also in þe ydropesie of þe moder, the chekys be nesshe & softe & febeliche ycoloured; but women with chyld ben oþerwhiles wel ycolered and her chekes harde & þer is gret difference. Also bytwene þe ydropesie of þe moder and wyndynesse of þe moder: For wyndes wyl liʒtliche vanysshe away; þe ydropesie wyl nought so. Also wyndes ben oþerwhile in þe tone side of þe moder & oþerwhile in þe other side but ydropesie occupieth all þe moder.

*gos oþer: MS. gosti.
† sanguinarie: MS. sanguarie.
‡ sanguinarie: MS. sanguarie.
§ empiricon: MS. ypericon.
**MS.: a blank line follows this sentence, instead of a chapter heading.
†† MS. margin: *Tokenes of chyde.*

drunk with the juice of artemisia does excellently; likewise, savory put in brings forth the dead child.

*Concerning an excessive discharge of blood.* Make a suppository of goose or goat's dung with the juice of knotgrass, apply it, and it staunches all bloody flux. So does a bath of plantain, the center bark of an oak tree, shepherd's rod, knotgrass, and other such empiricon, when drunk, staunch the flux of the womb.

For distress after childbirth: take yolks of egg boiled in water, ground wax, oil, juice of artemisia, powdered cinnamon, and make a plaster front and back, and immediately the suffering will cease. Also, if she has a fever, take onions boiled in water and mashed with the yolks of eggs boiled in water with oil and cumin powder, and make a plaster.

Dropsy of the uterus is sometimes due to a retention of the blood of which a woman should be purged, and then she cannot be healed until she is purged of that blood; sometimes the disease is due to wind and phlegmatic humors that are in the uterus, and then a woman swells with this dropsy as though she were pregnant. And there are many various signs to distinguish one from the other; for this swelling comes suddenly; the other dropsies do not. This swelling comes and goes, but the other stays always until a woman is delivered of a child; this dropsy moves from place to place, the other does not. Also, this dropsy moves indefinitely, while the other moves without question and at certain times in both the day and the night. But the [f. 212r] dropsy of the uterus, the movement and agitation, is frequently by night and seldom by day. Also, in dropsy of the uterus the cheeks are pliant, soft, and pale; but women with child have good coloring at other times, and their cheeks are firm, and there is a great difference. Also [there is a difference] between dropsy of the uterus and windiness of the uterus: for winds will pass easily away; the dropsy will not. Also, winds are sometimes on one side of the uterus and sometimes on the other, but dropsy takes up the whole of the uterus.

Also wyndes ben euermore within the moder and they may be withoute gret feblenesse of þe moder, that it ne is nouȝt myghti to defeye the fleumatik humours þat ben within her & sche may nouȝt put hem awey fro her.

*Cura*: for to helpen the moder of syknesse, it behouyth þat þe moder be purged of þe humours þat be within her & þat hathe be told here before bothe in þe precipitacion of þe moder and also in withholdyng of þe blode. Natheles, make her a stuphe of tyme, calamint, of origanum, of saveray, of lauendre, of rue, of puliol* riall & mountayn, of mugwede & of lorer leves & the croppes of hennebane, of comyn, carui, of smallache, loveache, chervyle, parcilie, stanmarche, of eueriche an handfull; let sethe hem in water & do stuphe her in þat sethyng of þo herbes also long as she may; and whan she goth out of þe stuphe, ley þe herbes to þe moder. A good suppositorie to purgen þe moder of suche fleumatik humours: Take þe floure of cokell & medled with hony & oyle & make hit sadde as paste is þat brede is made of and wynde it in a softe lynnen clothe & put it in her prevy mem-[f. 212v]bre. But teye it with a threde aboute her thyes lest þe moder drawe it in all to herre, & lete hit ligge there all a nyght oþer longer yf it nede. But first make a plaster of lekes grounde & fryed in her owne jus & ley it from her navell douneward to hir prevy membre & ouer it. On þe morew, yf þe moder smert withynforth of þe sharpnesse of þe cokell, anoynt it with oile of roses, oþer of violet, and with þe muscillage of dragantum made with þe jus of violet and þe white of an eye, & medle hem togedre & anoynt þe place therwith till it be hole. And ther was a woman in London & had this ydropesie & she was holden mourrable thorough all leches of that towne of London. But the woman toke & made her wortes with these herbes thorough her owne wytte. She toke waterkersis an handfull, of sowthistelis & southistelis of fen, of wylde sauge, of parcely, of beteyne, of millefoyle, of goldes, of euerich þe sixt parte of an handfull & made her wortes & ete herof al greene as moche as euer she myȝt susteyne & kept her from all drynkes saue from those wortes þat she ete of hem ayenst nyght ix sithes or x on a day instede of drynke, & yf she muste algates drynk, she drank this ptysan. Sche toke a dysshe-full of barly, of wormode, of rotes of stanmarche, of parcely, aneys seed, of fenel, of goldes, ambrose, of sowthistle & of scarliol ana *li*. i, & sethe all these in thre galons of clere water till þe

*puliol: MS. piliol.

Also, winds are always within the uterus, and they can be there without great impairment to the uterus, so that it is not advisable to break down the phlegmatic humors that are inside and cannot be expelled.

*Cure*: To heal the uterus of this sickness, it must be purged of the humors that are inside it, and the procedure has already been described here in connection with the precipitation of the uterus and the retention of blood. Nevertheless, make her a bath of a handful each of thyme, calamint, origanum, savory, lavender, rue, pennyroyal, wild thyme, artemisia, laurel leaves, and the sprigs of henbane, cumin, caraway, smallage, lovage, chervil, parsley, and horse-parsley; boil them in water and put her in a hot bath of those herbs for as long as she can stand it; and when she comes out of the bath, put the herbs on the uterus. A good suppository to purge the uterus of such phlegmatic humors: take cockle flour and mix it with honey and oil, and make as firm as bread dough, and wrap up the paste in a soft linen cloth and put it in her privy mem-[f. 212v]ber. But tie it with a thread about her thighs lest the uterus draw it entirely inside, and let it lie there all night or longer if necessary. But first make a plaster of leeks ground and fried in their own juice and place it from the navel down to her privy member and on top. The next day, if the uterus smarts inside because of the sharpness of the cockle, anoint it with oil of roses or violets and with the gum tragacanth made with the juice of violets and the white of an egg, and mix them together and anoint the place until it is healed. There was a woman in London who had this dropsy, and she was considered incurable by all the London doctors. But this woman took and made her pottage with these herbs, through her own common sense. She took a handful of watercresses, a sixth part of a handful each of sow thistles, marsh sow thistles, wild sage, parsley, betony, milfoil, and marigolds, and made pottage and ate it all fresh, as much as she could take. She abstained from all fluids except that from these herbs, which she ate nine times a night or ten times a day instead of fluid, and if she had to drink in any case, she drank this ptisan. She took a dishful of barley, 1 pound each of wormwood, roots of horse-parsley, parsley, anise seed, fennel, marigolds, wild sage, sow thistle, green endive, and boiled all these in 3 gallons of clear water until haluendel was consumed away & hereof she drank erliche & late, & she lete garsen her legges ouer all ayenst þe fyre & after she layd to her legges levis of clotes. And so she hadde wrapped her leggis in tho clote leves and it drow out [f. 213r] all that mischief, and she bathed her prevy membre with jus of puliol riall and with origanum and mugwede with a pipe & þeron was a bladder & she lete poure þe jussis into her wombe by her prevy membre. And she made a plaster of diptayne, of isop & of saueray and leid it to her prevy shappe withouteforth, and þis plastre brouȝt forth her priue termes and with þese medecines she was made hole. The bred þat she ete was this: Tak a pek of bene mele & do knede it with vynegre & lete bake it & ete of that brede in hir potage abouesaid. And she wisshe her body aboute þe lyver with þe jus of elf-hame.

*The 7 Chapiter is of the rawnesse that whan the moder semyth flayne.*

The moder semyth ofte flayne & rawe as a thyng þat were forscalded; that is whan kende colrik humours chawviþ and brennyth aboute þe moder withynforth. And þe signes & þe tokens herof ben brennynges and prikkinges & smertinges withynforth; and oþerwhiles þe moder is forblayned and scabbed withinforth of suche humours, and than she shal fele moche ichching withinforth.
*Cura*: to hele hem of þis greuaunce, lete purgen hem with þe electuarie de succo rosarum and sithe let make her a stuphe of colde herbes and afterward lete her blede on þe veyne vnder þe ancle withinforth of þe fote. And afterward, let tempre licium with cowe mylk & cast it into the moder with a pissarie, as men doth purgen a mannes wombe with a clistre þorough his fundament, and let caste in at one tyme þe quantite of a *li*. i, & lete her vsen this the thirde day that iche vnderstond [f. 213v] from thre daies to thre daies forto she be hole. Another pouder: take of þe seed of whyte popie & gumme arabik & dragaunte & spodie ana ȝ i, poudre hem with rayne water & make rounde balles of hem & whan it nedith, medle hem with cowe mylk & late vnderfonge þerof with a pissorie at hir prevy membre. Also anoynt it withynforth with þe marye of a calfe oþer with fresshe butter other with summe other suche fresshe thyng, and in clensyng of þe moder for corupt humours, bewarre þer come no violent thyng in her, lest þou make þe woman bareyn so ever. But

half of it was evaporated. And she drank this all the time, and she had her legs scarified all over by the fire and afterward she put burdock leaves on her legs. And so she wrapped her legs in those burdock leaves, and it drew out [f. 213r] all that trouble, and she bathed her privy member in the juice of pennyroyal, origanum, artemisia, using a pipe to which a bladder was attached, and she got the juice poured into her womb through her privy member. And she made a plaster of dittany, hyssop, savory, and placed it on her private parts externally, and this plaster brought on her menstrual periods, and with these medicines she was cured. The bread that she ate was this: take a peck of bean meal, knead it with vinegar, have it baked, and eat that bread with the pottage described above. And she washed her body around the liver with hellebore juice.

*The seventh chapter is concerned with the rawness that occurs when the uterus seems to be excoriated.*

The uterus often seems to be excoriated and raw as though it were scalded. This occurs when the natural choleric humors consume and burn about the uterus inside. And the signs and symptoms of this ailment are burnings, prickings, and smartings inside; and sometimes the womb is blistered and scabbed inside by such humors, and then she feels much itching inside.

*Cure:* To cure women of this complaint, have them purge themselves with the electuary of rose juice, and afterwards have the patient make a bath of cold herbs, and then bleed her on the vein under the ankle inside the foot. And afterward mix licium* with cow's milk and throw it into the womb with a pessary, just as one purges a man's stomach with an enema through the anus, and throw in 1 pound at a time and if she uses this the third day, so I understand it, [f. 213v] and every third day, she will be cured. Another powder: take 1 ounce each of white poppy seed, gum arabic, gum tragacanth, and slag, powder them with rainwater, make round balls of them and, when necessary, mix with cow's milk, and let her receive the medicament with a pessary in her privy member. Also, oil it inside with the marrow of a calf, fresh butter, or some other fresh thing, and in cleansing the uterus of corrupt humors, see that nothing too strong is put in her, lest you make the woman barren forever. But

* A medicinal powder made from dried juice of certain plants [*M.E.D.*].

vse these þingis in pissaries þat mowe comfort þe moder. And if þe woman be poure, than sethe moleyn & þe barke of sloue trees in tanwater, & whan they ben well soden, lete hir sitte theryn vp to þe navell, & whan þat she is wery, reyse hir from þat bath & make her this smokyng: Take rose leves, clowes, frankencense, mirr ana ʒ i, & brose hem togeder, & whan all this is done, þanne caste þat poudre on small coles & lete hir sitte a while ther over. Or els take mastik ℈ i, bole armoniak, terra sigillata, wormeton, pouder of oke tre that no lyme comyth nygh, sangdragon ana ℈ i, litargii aurei ʒ ii, poudre all these riȝt small & lete a priue woman cast it there that þe rawnesse is, & this poudre shal hele it &cetera.

*The 8 Chapiter is of þe apostumes of the moder þat is full sore.*

Apostume of þe moder comyth in diuerse parties of þe moder; otherwhiles in þe innermest partie of þe moder and oþerwhiles in þe mouthe of þe moder. Yf it be clene in þe depnesse of þe moder, she felith ache from [f. 214r] the mydryf to þe prevy membre, and her sides swellyne; & they haue greuaunce to brethen & to drawe wynde also. But þe grettest greuaunce that thei haven is abouten her share & her raynes. And this enpostume comyth oþerwhiles of hote humours and oþerwhiles of cold. Yf it is of blode, þer is ache & prikkyng þere as þe mater of þe enpostume is gadered* togedre & they haue continually a continuall fever, butt noȝt to stronge, & þe veynes of her legges swellen. Her vryne is clere rede, and oþerwhiles dym rede, & a maner of swart rede abouen vnder þe cercle. Yf it be of colre, þat is, an hote humour & drye, she hath these forsaid tokens, but they be more violent þan ben blody tokens: the vryn is moche thynne, full citrine, the pousse riȝt swyft, þe maladie in þe riȝt side for the galle where his dominion stant. Yif it is a colde humour & a moiste, she felith bothe greuaunce & hevynesse in þe moder, & her vryn is trobely & febelich ycoloured & of þe colour of axen vnder þe cercle. Yf it be of melancolie þat is a colde humour & drie, sche hath moche heuynesse in þe moder and þe veynes of her legges ben of swart yelowe colour of lede and þei fallen in an esy fever. But whan þer

*gadered: MS. genderd.

use these things in pessaries that may comfort the uterus. And if the woman is poor, then boil mullein and the bark of blackthorn trees in tanning water, and when they have been well boiled, let her sit in the solution up to her navel. When she is weary, lift her from the bath and make this fumigation: take 1 drachm each of rose leaves, cloves, frankincense, and myrrh, mash them together, and when this is done cast powder on small coals, and let her sit over it for a while. Or else take 1 scruple each of mastic, Armenian bole, Lemnian earth, wormwood, powder from an oak tree that has had no lime on it, sandragon, 2 drachms of litharge of gold, powder all these very small, and let a discreet woman put it where the rawness is, and this powder will heal it, etc.

*The eighth chapter is concerned with inflammations of the uterus that is very sore.*

Inflammation of the uterus occurs in various parts of it; sometimes it is in the innermost part of the uterus and sometimes at the mouth of it. If it is right in the depth of the uterus, the woman feels an ache from [f. 214r] the midriff to the privy member, and her sides swell; and women have difficulty in breathing and in getting their wind also. But the greatest discomfort that they have is about their private parts and their kidneys. And this inflammation comes sometimes from hot humors and sometimes from cold. And if it is due to the blood, there is aching and pricking where the matter of the inflammation has gathered together, and women have an incessant mild fever and the veins of their legs swell. Their urine is bright red, and sometimes dull red, and a kind of dark redness appears under the opening of the anus. If it be of bile, that is, a hot, dry humor, she has the previously mentioned signs, but they are more violent than are the tokens due to the blood: the urine is very thin, bright yellow, the pulse is very swift, the sickness is on the right side, because the hot humor has its dominion in the gall bladder. But if it is due to a cold, moist humor, she feels both discomfort and heaviness in the uterus, and her urine is cloudy, poorly colored, and of the color of ashes under the opening of the anus. And if it is due to melancholy, which is a cold, dry humor, she has much heaviness in the uterus and the veins of her legs are the dark yellow color of lead, and such women fall into a mild fever. But when there is

is a postume in þe moder & the vryn is whyte & thynne, þat is a
feble signe for to help. For to help of þat sekenesse, fyrst lete hym
bleden at þe veyne vnder þe ancle; and afterward, in þe first
begynnyng of þe enpostume, þou muste vsen colde plasters þat
ben repercussiues to driue þe maters ayenwarde. As make a
plaster of þe innest pelyng of hempe & of þe jus of pety morell
warmed, & ley that to þe enpostume a twyes or thryes and
remene a day. [f. 214v] Also anoynt the wombe ayen the enpostume with oile of roses oþer of violet. And yf þe enpostume
be of hete & of hote humours, lete her eten colde herbes as
partulake, letuse, & endyve & suche oþer, & drynk þe water þat
is distilled of suche herbes. Afterward, than whan þe enpostume
is full ywoxen, make emplasters to make it to wexe & to ripe &
nesshe to breke; as is a plastre þat is made of wete mele soden in
oile oþer in fresshe butter & a litell water. Other make a plaster of
mele of lynesede oþer of fenugrek* medled with lye, but lete
nout þat lye be full stronge. Oþer medle suche stronge lye with†
barly mele & make þerof a plastre. Oþer take oyle comune, sowre
dowȝ, fresshe butter oþer grece, jus of merche ana ℥ ii, lynesede,
fenugrek ana ℥ i & sem., bismalowe ysperate ℥ iii, water of
snayles ℥ sem.; sethe all these togeder, probatum est. But yf þe
enpostume come of colde humours, gyf hir þe sirup þat is made
of fenell rotes, of parcely, & of merche with her sedes & of dauke
& carui, radich, enula campana, zuccre water & hony as moche
as nedith. And in þe beginning also of þis enpostume, make her
emplasters of origanum, of ysope, of centorie, of rue, & of
celidonye ana ℥ i, sode in wyne oþer in water & layd to all warme.
Afterward whan þe enpostume is full woxen, make enplastres to
make þe enpostume ripe; oon is this: take whete mele & oyle of
violet & hony & make þerof a plastre. Anoþer, make a plaster of
snayles soden in hony with whete mele oþer with mele made of
lynesede. Oþer make a plaster of þe rotes of affodille stamped, &
reysyns & fygges that ben drie, soden with lye & with wyne &
with [f. 215r] oyle. Oþer make a plastre of soure dowe soden in
oile; oþer a plaster of rue soden with wyne & with oile; oþer of
fenel sede, oþer of merche, oþer of rue ystamped and soden with
oile. And lete anoynte her with hote oynementis, as with dewte

*fenugrek: MS. femygrek.
† with: MS. with with.

an inflammation in the uterus, and the urine is white and thin, that is a slight indication that help is necessary. To help that complaint, first have her bled at the vein under the ankle; and afterward, at the very beginning of the abscess, you must use cold plasters, which are repellents to drive the matters away. For this, make a plaster of the innermost layer of hemp, and the juice of black nightshade warmed, and place that on the inflammation twice or thrice, remaining there for a day. [f. 214v] Anoint the uterus for an inflammation with oil of roses or violet. And if the inflammation is hot and of hot humors, let her eat cold herbs such as purslane, lettuce, endive, and other similar herbs, and drink water that is distilled from such herbs. Afterward, when the abscess is fully developed, prepare plasters to make it grow and ripen and become soft enough to break; such a plaster is one made of wheat meal boiled in oil or fresh butter and a little water. Alternatively, make a plaster of meal with linseed or fenugreek mixed with lye, but see that the lye is not very strong. Or mix strong lye with barley meal and make a plaster of it. Or take 2 drachms each of common oil, sour dough, fresh butter or fat, and celery juice, 1½ drachms of linseed and fenugreek, 3 drachms of marshmallow separated, half a drachm of juice of snails; boil all these together; the prescription has been proven to be effective. But if the inflammation is the result of cold humors, give her syrup that is made of fennel roots, parsley, celery with its seeds, wild carrot, caraway, radish, horseheal, sugar water, and honey, as much as is necessary. And at the start also of this inflammation, make her plasters of 1 drachm each of origanum, hyssop, centaury, rue, and celandine, boiled in wine or water and laid on warm. Afterward, when the abscess has fully developed, prepare plasters to make it ripe; one is this: take wheat meal, oil of violet, honey, and make a plaster of them. Or make a plaster of snails boiled in honey with wheat meal or with meal made from linseed. Or make a plaster of the crushed roots of asphodel, and raisins and figs that are dried, boiled with lye, wine, and [f. 215r] oil. Or make a plaster of sour dough boiled in oil; or a plaster of rue boiled in wine and oil; or of fennel seed, celery, or rue, crushed and boiled with oil. And see that she is anointed with hot ointments, such as deute* and

---

* A kind of salve made from milfoil, catmint, henbane, and other ingredients.

& with marciaton. Oþer thinges þer ben full goode to make þe enpostume rype, as þe grece of hennys & of ganders & þe marie of an herte, other of a calfe & rede wex & oile of roses & womannes mylk & þe white of an eye; they be goode bothe to plastre withouten & ben profitable also to ben receyed withinforth thorough a pissorie atte þe prevy membre. And whan þe enpostume is tobroken, thou shalt knowe it by þe quyttour & þe corupcion þat comyth away þerfrom. Take þan meeth & warme yt ℥ xxii, & do þerto ℥ vii of clene hony, & lete here receyue þerof þe quantite of ℥ xvi þorough* a pissarie to make þe moder clene. Oþer take the oþer medecynes þat weren ytold in þe nexte chapeter.

*The 9 Chapiter ys of akyng of the moder.*

Ache of þe moder comyth oþerwhile of a dede bore chylde that is bore rather than his tyme. Wherfore þe moder hath a grete likyng & a comfort of þe chylde þat is within her, and whan she lesith it she makith a kendeliche mornyng & a sorewyng riȝt as a kowe doth whan she hath lost her calf, & that sorewyng is ache of þe moder. And oþerwhile þe moder akith for colde; & oþerwhile for hete, but þat nys but selde. Yf it be of colde þer is ache & prikking in þe left side & oþer tokens that have be tolde be-[f. 215v]fore. And herefore take pulioll riall, origanum, lorer leves, calamynt, & hokkes, and sethe hem in water & in wyne, and þerwith wasshe her wombe from þe navell doun to hir prevy membre. Sithen take clowes, spycenarde, notemuges, galingale & make her a fumygacion bynetheforth. Or els take mirr, olibanum, origanum, calamynt, cipresse, anise, & make a fumigacion. Oþer, take laudanum for fumigacion. Oþer thinges also þat I haue tolde here before ben good for the ache of þe moder wheder it be of cold or of hete. But for the ache of þe moder þat comyth after þat a woman hathe borne a childe, take rue & mugwede & wormode ana *m*. i, camphor ℥ ii, stampe hem & pouder þe camphor & sethe hem in oyle of puliole & hete it wel ayenst þe fyre & wrappe it in a clothe from þe navell douneward. Also for ache þat comyth of hardnesse of þe moder, take saxifrage & groundswelly & of olde cowle & mugwede & hokkes & betayne & sethe hem wel in

*þorough: MS. þorouhg.

marciation.* Other things that are very effective in making an abscess ripe are hen's and gander's fat, the marrow of a hart or calf, red wax, oil of roses, woman's milk, and the white of egg; these are good for a plaster on the outside and are also effective when taken inside through a pessary at the privy member. And when the abscess is broken, you will know by the purulent discharge and pus that comes away from it. Then take 22 drachms of mead, warm it, add to it 7 drachms of clear honey, and let her take in the amount of 16 ounces through a pessary to cleanse the uterus. Or take the different medicines that were described in the adjoining chapter.

*The ninth chapter is concerned with aching of the uterus.*

Ache of the uterus is sometimes due to a stillborn child being born before his time. Because the mother has great contentment and happiness from the child inside her, when she loses it she naturally mourns and grieves just as a cow does when she has lost her calf, and that distress causes the ache of the uterus. And sometimes the uterus aches because of cold; and sometimes because of heat, but that is rare. If it is due to cold there is aching and pricking on the left side and other signs that have already been described. [f. 215v] And for this take pennyroyal, origanum, laurel leaves, calamint, and mallows, boil them in water and wine, and wash her womb with the liquid from the naval down to her privy member. Afterward take cloves, spikenard, nutmegs, galingale, and make her a fumigation down below. Or else take myrrh, olibanum, origanum, calamint, cypress, anise, and make a fumigation. Or take ladanum† for fumigation. Other things also that I have described previously are good for the ache of the uterus, whether it is due to coldness or heat. But for the ache of the uterus that comes after a woman has given birth to a child, take 1 handful each of rue, artemisia, and wormwood, and 2 ounces of camphor, mash them, powder the camphor, and boil them in oil of thyme. Heat well on the fire and wrap in a cloth from the navel downward. Also for aching due to the hardness of the uterus, take saxifrage, groundsel, old cabbage, artemisia, mallows, and betony, and boil them well in

* A kind of ointment frequently recommended for aching bones and joints.
† A resin obtained from a plant of the genus *cistus*. Not to be confused with the laudanum of the sixteenth century.

water, & lete þe woman sitte in þat water vp to þe tetes. And whan she comyth out þerof, make a plastre of hokkis & of wormode & of camphor stamped togeder with oyle of puliole oþer of lorer & sithe hette ouer þe fyre & ley it on þe moder. For þe same: take þe leves of herbe þat is cleped baume *m*. ii, wormode, hokkis ana *m. sem.*, grynde hem with a litell white wyne & oyle de Bay & hete it & leye it on as is beforesaid. Oþerwhiles whan þe woman is deliuerd of childe, þe moder walkith in þe wombe from oon place to anoþer & akith for also moche as she is sodenly emptid of þe child and made her fulle before. And for þis sekenesse take þe croppes of ellerne & stampe hem & wrynge oute þe jus [f. 216r] & þerwith & with eyren & with whete mele, make her thynne cakes & frye hem so in fresshe grece & that schall sese þe ache. And gyve hyr warme wyne to drynke þat comyn was soden yn.

*Iff þou wylt knowe wel & trewly whether a woman be with chyld oþer none withoute lokyng of water.*

Yff a woman be with childe, take hyr to drynke mede whan she shal wende to bedde. And yf she haue moche wo in her wombe, it is a signe þat she is with childe. Also yf þe trociscis of mirre as Rasis saith with water that juniperii ben soden yn & after that they be ydronke, yf she be with retencion of his floures than is riȝt grete sorowe folewyng. And also they casten out a dede childe. And þe cause is for þe trociscis makyn sotill & viscous mater. Also they open & they beten the marice, and also they strengthen þe vertue expulsef* & þerfore þei ben good. Also þe thingis þat shall casten out a dede childe from þe marice, they muste be myȝttyer þan tho that helpen to haue esy birthe. The thingis þat helpen to haue forth a dede child fro þe marice ben thre thingis: The first is galbanum ℥ ii resolued in gotis mylk that þe woman may esely vsen a two ounces of þe melke oþer thre. The seconde is to make a suppositorie thus: R℞: ollis nigri, stafizacre, aristolochia rotunda, bothon,† morien, granorum lauriole, pulpe colloquintide, gummi armoniaci ana ℥ ii, fel bouis ℥ i; make pouder, saue of gummi aromatici, resolue it in jus arthemesie with þe whiche medle alle the oþer pouders & make a suppositorie. Or els with more of fel bouis and of þe jus of arthemesie make a pissorie with a litell oyle. Also a plaster þat [f.

*expulsef: MS. expulseth.
† bothon: MS. bothor.

water, and let the woman sit in that water up to her nipples. And when she comes out of it, make a plaster of mallows, wormwood, camphor, crushed together with oil of wild thyme or laurel, and afterward heat it over the fire and place it on the womb. For the same: take 2 handfuls of the leaves of the herb that is called balm, and half a handful each of wormwood and mallows, mash them with a little white wine and oil of bay, heat it, and lay it on as previously described. Sometimes when a woman has given birth to a child the uterus moves in the belly from one place to another, and aches inasmuch as the woman is suddenly emptied of the child that previously made her full. And for this sickness, take the shoots of sambucus, bruise them, wring out the juice, [f. 216r] and with the juice, eggs, and wheat meal, make her thin cakes and fry them in fresh fat, and that will stop the aching. And give her warm wine to drink in which cumin has been boiled.

*If you would establish with certainty whether a woman is pregnant or not without examining the urine.*

If a woman is pregnant, get her to drink mead when she goes to bed. And if she has much discomfort in her belly, it is a sign that she is with child. Also pills of myrrh, as Rhazes says, taken with water that juniper has been boiled in, cause great distress after they are drunk, if the woman is not menstruating. And also they cast out a dead child. And the reason for this is that the pills make thin and gluey matter. Also, they open and relieve the womb, strengthen the body's natural ability to eliminate toxics, and therefore they are good. Further, the things that cast out a dead child from the womb must be more powerful than those that assist in making childbirth easy. The things that help to bring out a dead child from the womb are three. The first is 2 drachms of galbanum dissolved in goat's milk, so that the woman can easily take 2 or 3 ounces of the milk. The second is to make a suppository thus: take 2 drachms each of black olive oil, stavesacre, round birthwort, rosemary, marjoram, the seeds of laurel, the succulent part of colocynth, and gum ammoniac, and 1 drachm of bull's gall; reduce to powder, with the exception of the aromatic resin, dissolve in the juice of artemisia, then mix with it all the other ingredients and make a suppository. Alternatively, with more of the bull's gall and the juice of artemisia, make a pessary with a little oil. Another plaster that

216v] castith out a dede childe fro the marice, oon þerof is this: take galbanum *li. sem.* & tempre it with þe jus of mugwede & ley it on a lether in quantite of a pawme & two fyngers more in lengthe, in brede of a litell pawme & ley it vnder þe navell toward þe prevy membre. Anoþer: take þe jus of rue *li. sem.*, mirre poudred ℥ iiii, pouder of colloquintide ℥ iii & encorpore hem togeder in a nesshe maner; make a plaster & warme ley it to vnder the navel on þe wombe. Also to haue esy byrthe of þe childe, take ℥ vi of þe barke off cassiefistule & drynke it with wyne oþer with þe broth of rede chiches. Anoþer: take azari, castorei ana ℥ ii sotelliche pouderd, & yeve it with decoccion of rede chiches. The third is as Auicen seith: take mirre, castorei, storacis, calaminte ana ℥ *sem.*, inward barke of canell ychosen, saveyn ana Ə *sem.*, make pouder, & yeve it hir whan she trauayleth of child with a litel hony & it helpith moche to de-liueren þe child and þe secundine. Anoþer thing is necessarie: that is þat her knees ben bounden to her navel & that she be put in a short place, & than gyve hyr vomites, for it helith moche. Also take agrimoyne with his rotis & lay the rotes toward þe marice, & whan she childith do it away lest þe marice folowe. And þis experiment, tellen all þe doctours, yf God wyll hit helpith moche to haue chylde.

*The 10 Chapiter is of þe greuaunces þat wommen haue in beryng of her chyldren.*

Greuaunces þat women haue in bering of her children comyth in two maners, that is to say kyndely & vnkyndely. Whan it is kyndelich, þe chyld comyth forth with-[f. 217r]in a xx$^{ti}$ throwes or withyn tho twenty, & the child comyth in fourme as it shuld: first þe heved & sithen þe nek & with þe armes & shulders & with his oþer membres fourmeabely as it shuld. And also in þe se-conde maner, þe chyld comyth forth vnkyndely, & þat may be in 16 maners as ye shuld fynde in hyr propre chapiters, and fyrst thus.

Whan þe childes hede aperith, as it were, hedelinges, and all þe oþer partie of þe chyld levith in þe moder syde: the help herof is that þe mydwif with her honde anoynted in oyles, id est, in oyle of pulioll & in oyle of lilie merue* or oyle muscelleum and, as it nedith, that honde so anoynted and put in & fourmabely dress-yng þe child with her hondes from þe sides of þe moder. And þe

*merue: MS. mesue.

[f. 216v] expels a dead child from the womb is this: take half a pound of galbanum, mix it with the juice of artemisia, and spread it on the piece of leather, the size of your palm and two fingers in length and a small palm in breadth, and place it under the navel near the privy member. Another: take half a pound of juice of rue, 4 drachms of powdered myrrh, and 3 drachms of colocynth, and mix them gently together; make a plaster and put it warm under the navel on the womb. Also, to promote easy childbirth, take 6 ounces of the bark of cassia fistula and drink it with wine or with the broth of red chick-peas. Another: take 2 drachms each of hazelwort, and dried beaver-gland carefully powdered, and give with a preparation of boiled red chick-peas. The third is as Avicenna says: take half a drachm each of myrrh, dried beaver-gland, gum, and calamint, half a scruple each of the inside bark of choice cinnamon and savin, make a powder, and give this medicament to her with a little honey when she is in labor, and it greatly assists the delivery of the child and the secundine. Another thing is necessary: that is, that her knees be held close to her navel and that she should be put in a contracted space, and then give her emetics, for they are very helpful. Also, take agrimony with its roots and lay the roots toward the womb, and when she has given birth, take it away lest the womb follow. And this experiment, according to all the doctors, greatly assists in childbirth, if God wills.

*The tenth chapter is concerned with the sicknesses that women have in childbearing.*

Sicknesses that women have bearing children are of two kinds, natural and unnatural. When it is natural, the child comes out [f. 217r] in twenty pangs or within those twenty, and the child comes the way it should: first the head, and afterward the neck, and with the arms, shoulders, and other members properly as it should. In the second way, the child comes out unnaturally, and that may be in sixteen ways, as you will find in their proper chapters, and the first is as follows:

When the child's head appears, as it were, head first, and the rest of the child remains inside the uterus. The remedy for this is that the midwife, with her hand anointed with oils, that is, wild thyme oil, pure lily oil, or oil of musk, as is necessary, put her hand in and turn the child properly with her hands from the sides of the uterus. And [see that]

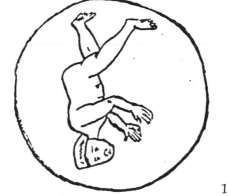

1

Reproductions of the birth figures from this manuscript, Sloane 2463, illustrating the various malpositions the midwife is to correct.

orifice of þe marice so anoynted well þat þe childe may come forth evenly. The seconde maner is vnkyndely also, whan þe childe comyth with his feete joyntly togeder, but the mydwyf shall never haue it forth whan he comyth so douneward. But when he begynnyth to come so to, þe mydwiff with her handes anoynted & yn put shove hym vp ayen & dresse hym so þat he may come forth on þe moste kyndely maner þat he sqwat nouȝt his hondes in þe moder sides. The third maner vnkyndely is yf þe childes hede be so moche & so grete that he may not come forth: [f. 217v] the mydwyf than schal shove hym ayen & anoynt with may butter that is fresshe or with oyle comune þe orifice, id est, þe mouthe of þe prive membre, & þan þe mydwifys honde put in so anoynted first, and that membre made large, than brynge hym forth holding þe hed of hym.

The 4 maner yf þe child come forth ayenst kynde, she that trauaylith schall be brouȝt into a schort strayte bedde that hath an hygh stondyng and sche put out her hede, than the mydwif hauyng her hond anoynted and put yn after þat it is vnkyndeliche & ydressed hym rightlich & þan so brynge hym forth; but þe bedde þat þe woman schall lyggen yn schuld be made harde.

The 5 manere ayenst kynde ys yf þe child proferth his hande first forth & his hede be turned ayen & the mouthe of þat priue membre be streyte or schytte; thanne, with that constreynyng of þe handes of þe mydwyf, that thilk way be larged and þat þe childis hande be put in ayen þat þe child be nouȝt slayne

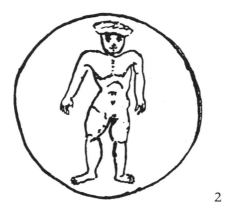

2

the orifice of the womb is so well anointed that the child can come forth in right order.

The second mode of unnatural childbirth occurs when the child comes out with his feet jointly together, only the midwife can never bring the child out when it comes down like this. But when the child begins to come out in this way, the midwife with her hands anointed with oil must put them in and push him up again and so arrange him that he can come forth in the most natural manner, so that he does not flatten his hands in the sides of the uterus.

The third unnatural mode is if the child's head is so bulky and large that he cannot emerge: [f. 217v] the midwife should then push him back and anoint the orifice, that is, the mouth of the privy member with fresh May butter or with common oil, and then the midwife's hand, oiled first and then put in and the orifice enlarged, brings the child forth by the head.

In the fourth mode of unnatural childbirth, the woman in labor shall be placed in a short, narrow, high-standing bed, with her head off the bed, and the midwife, with her hand anointed with oil, thrusts her hand in after the child who is in an unnatural position, turns him correctly, and then brings him forth; but the bed that the woman should lie in must be made hard.

The fifth mode of unnatural childbirth is when the child extends his hand first, his head is turned back, and the mouth of the privy member is narrow or shut; then, with the inducement of the hands of the midwife, the orifice should be enlarged, and the child's hand put in again so that the child does not die as the

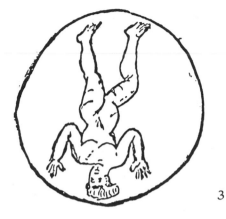

3

þoroughe þe mydwifes defaute. We comaunde þe mydwifes honde putte in, dressynge þe childes schuldres to be put bakwardes & her hondes riȝtlyche dressed to her sides. And than þe hed of þe child take; than so lete brynge hym forth.

The 6 maner ayenst kynde is yf þe childe profer forth his bothe hondes with his two schulderis [f. 218r], and settyng his two handis þat oon on þat oon side & þe other on þat oþer side, and þe hed is turned bakward into þe side ayenward. The mydwyf with her honde schall put hym ayen as we saide in þe next chapiter, that is, sche schal dresse his hondes to his sydes and take childes hede & esely bryng hym forthe. Yf he haue a litell hede & his hondis, yf he caste first outward, the mydwyf schall ordeyne þat þe hede may come to þe mouth of þe priue membre, & so by hyr handes she shall bryng hym forth by þe grace of God.

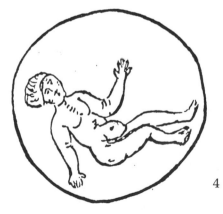

4

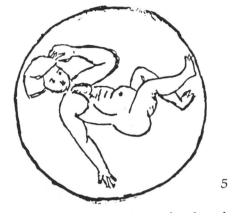

5

result of the midwife's error. We prescribe that the midwife put her hand in, turning the child's shoulders toward the back and hands properly down at the side. And then take the head of the child; then slowly bring him forth.

The sixth mode of unnatural childbirth is when the child extends both his hands with his two shoulders, [f 218r] with his hands one on one side and one on the other, and the head is turned back in a reversed position into the side. The midwife with her hand shall put the child in again, as we said in the adjoining chapter, that is, she should put his hands to his sides, take the child's head, and gently bring him forth. If he has a small head, and if he throws out his hands first, the midwife should arrange for the head to come to the mouth of the privy member, and so by her hands she shall bring him forth by the grace of God.

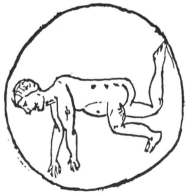

6

128

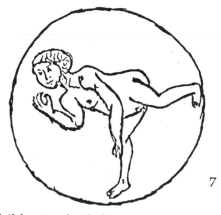

7

The 7 is yf þe child caste forth fyrste his right foot, the mydwiff schal neuer bryng hym forth so, but sche shall fyrst sette hyr fyngers and put it vp ayenward; and after þat, sche schall putt yn honde & amende þat fote with þat oþer fote so corect hem bothe togeders yf it may be & his hondes to his sides & his fete so as þay out to ben, & so bryng hym forth.

The 8 is yf þe childe put forthe boþe feet & þe toþer dele of þe childe left in þe body bowande as we said first. The mydwyf with hyr honde yshoven yn & she besiliche dressyng þe chylde and so bryng hym forthe as I said abouen.

The 9 is yf þe childe schewe fyrst oon honde & oon foot & with þe tother honde he helith his face.

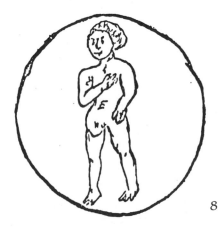

8

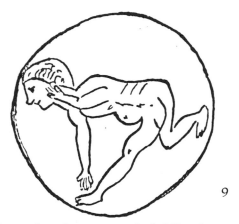

9

The seventh mode of unnatural childbirth occurs when the child first throws out his right foot, and the midwife will never deliver him in this way unless she first applies her fingers and puts the child up again; and after that, she must put in her hand and align that foot with the other foot to get both feet in the right position if possible, and the child's hands to his sides, and his feet as they should be, and then bring the child forth.

The eighth mode of unnatural childbirth occurs when the child puts out both feet and the rest of the child is left bent up in the body, as we said previously. The midwife with her hand shoved in should carefully arrange the child, and so bring him out, as I said previously.

The ninth mode of unnatural childbirth occurs when the child displays first one hand and one foot and covers his face with the other hand.

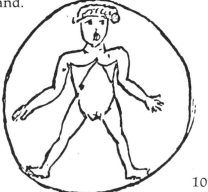

10

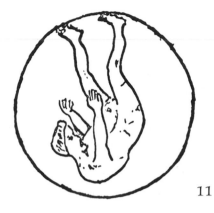

11

The mydwyf settyng hyr fyngers of hyr oon honde in þe grynde of þe woman þat trauaylith, [f. 218v] and with þe tother honde put it vp ayen as we haue schewid afore, & so bryng hym forth yf þou mayst.

The 10 is yf þe child schewe first forth his fete departyng and his oon honde bytwene his fete & his hede hangyng bakward. The mydwif with hyr honde putte in, correctyng þe chyld & leying hys oon honde by his other downe by his sides & mendyng his hede on þe best maner & þe feete rightlich dressed & than þe mydwif bryngyng hym forth.

The 11 is yf þe childes nekke come first foreward; than þe mydwiff hyr honde putte yn & shoue hym vp ayen by the shulders, highyng lyft the chyld & so to þe orificium bryng hym

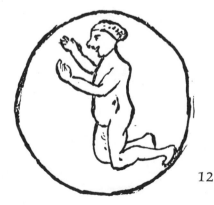

12

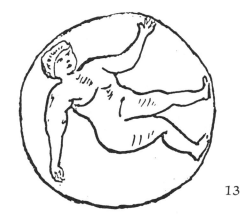

13

The midwife places the fingers of one hand on the groin of the woman in labor, [f. 218v] and with the other hand puts the child in again, as we have demonstrated before, and so brings the child forth if possible.

The tenth mode of unnatural childbirth occurs when the child presents first his feet apart, one hand between his feet, and his head hanging backward. The midwife with her hand put inside should correct the position of the child, placing one hand by the other down at his sides, adjusting the head in the best way, arranging the feet properly, and then bring the child forth.

The eleventh mode of unnatural childbirth occurs when the child's neck comes out first; then the midwife with her hand should push him up again by the shoulders, raise the child aloft, bring him

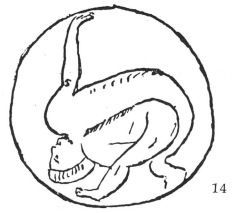

14

132

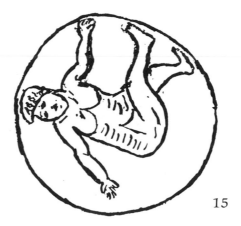

15

doune & so bryng him forth.

The 12 is yf þe child shewe fyrst forthe his knees bowed; than þe mydwiff schall put hym vp ayen bakward; the hondes of þe mydwif sette on oþer in hir gryndes and þan hir oon honde anoynded & put yn & þerwith amendyng so þe knees. And hym take by þe schulders & so bakward softely bryng hym forth. And so, whan his fete be amendid puttyng hym vpward vnto he be right as he schuld be & than bryng hym forth by the grace of God & þe mydwifes connyng.

The 13 is yf þe child schewe first forth his thyes & his comyng forth so erselyng; than þe mydwif with hyr honde put yn ayen by þe fete, she shal [f. 219r] brynge hym to þe orifice and evyn haue hym forth.                                                                                                      ·

The 14 is yf þe childes hede & þe soles of his fete come togeder; we bydde þan þe mydwif into þat prevye membre her hondes inshove & he taken & borne vp into þe wombe ayenward; than þe childe taken by þe hede & brought forthe.

The 15 is yf þe child lyeth grovelyng or els vpriȝt & his feete & his handes vpward abouen his hede; þan þe mydwif with hir fyngers put yn & þe child evenyd; þan, inasmoche as she may, lete þe hede come foreward & so bryng hym forthe.

The 16 is yf þer wer moo than oon, as it happith alday, & alle tho

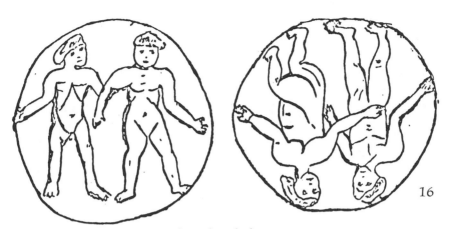

16

down to the orifice, and so fetch him out.

The twelfth mode of unnatural childbirth occurs when the child first presents his knees bent; then the midwife shall push him back in again; the midwife should put her hands on both sides in the woman's groin and then, with her own hand anointed with oil put inside, correct the position of the knees. And she should take the child by the shoulders and so gently bring him out backward. And so, when the position of his feet has been corrected and he has been put up in the right position, then bring him forth by the grace of God and the midwife's skill.

The thirteenth mode of unnatural childbirth occurs when the child first presents his thighs and comes forth with his buttocks first; then the midwife with her hand should put the child in again by the feet, and then [f. 219r] bring him to the orifice, and deliver him smoothly.

The fourteenth mode of unnatural childbirth is if the child's head and the soles of his feet come together; we instruct the midwife in such circumstances to push her hand into the privy member so that the child be taken and carried upward into the womb again; then the child should be grasped by the head and brought out.

The fifteenth mode of unnatural childbirth occurs when the child lies prostrate or else upright, and his feet and his hands are over his head. Then the midwife with her hand inside should straighten the child with her fingers; then, as far as she can, let the head come forward, and so bring the child out.

The sixteenth mode of unnatural childbirth occurs when there is more than one child, as happens every day, and they all be comyng to þe orifice at ones; than lete þe mydwyf putte ayen oon with hyr fyngers the whiles she hathe forth oon of þe children. And þan after, another, so doyng þat þe moder be noȝt repressed, noþer þe children mysfaren with all, as it fareth often tyme.

For to delyueren a woman of childe & for to sle it yf it may nought be brought forth: Take rue, saveyn, sothernewode, & gladon & lete hyr drynk hit. And also take þe jus of ysope, of dyptayn ana ȝ ii, quyksyluer Ӡ ii, & this medecyn is proved. Also take þe jus of yreos, of boles galle ana ȝ iiii, of mete oyle ȝ ii, medle all these togeders & do it in a pissorie & serve þe woman þerwith, & this medecyne will deliueren alle corupcions of þe marice. And it deliuereth hyr of a dede chyld & it wyl deliuere hyr of hir secundines & hit bryngith forth his menstruis. Item: da pregnangti ȝ ii asefetide, ter in die & vngantur* venter & dorsum cum oleo & felle, & postea ponantur oleum & fell bovis,† asefetide, in uuluis cum pluma. [f. 219v]

And þe greuaunces þat women hauen in beryng of children comyth otherwhiles of þe greuaunce of þe childe, & þat may be for þe childe is wel ywoxen in his moder wombe tofore sche hathe kaught þe ydropesye; and þis þe mydwif may wel knowe, and þe woman also. And oþerwhiles it comyth þorough þe feblenesse of þe moder þat sche nys noght myghty to putten þe childe oute from hyr. And þis may be in two maners: as for gret sekenesse that the woman hathe hadde & þat hathe febled hyr moche; or for gret thought of þe woman and yf she conceyued in þe fyrst of þe twelueyeres. Oþerwhiles it comyth of þe stoppyng of þe marice. And þat may be in two maners: as of fatnesse þat stoppith þe mouthe of þe marice & þat withholdith þe blode þat she shuld haue ben purged of er þat they hadde ben conceyued; or oþerwhiles it comyth for þe chyld is dede in his moder wombe. And tokens þer ben: oone is þat þei fele no steryng nor mevyng of þe chylde withynforth; anoþer is þe secunde day of hir trauaylyng, hyre mouthe stynketh; and another is þat þei felen gret ache & greuaunce aboute hir navell; anoþer is dissolucion of hir face & of all hir body; anoþer is þat þey desyren thynges that ben

*vngantur: MS. vngatus.
† bovis: MS. vocatur.

come to the orifice at once; then let the midwife put one back again with her fingers while she brings out one of the children. And then afterward, another, so doing that the uterus is not constricted nor the children brought to grief, as often happens.

In order to deliver a woman of a child and to kill it if it cannot be brought out: take rue, savin, southernwood, and iris, and let her drink them. Also take 2 drachms each of the juice of hyssop, and of dittany, and 2 scruples of quicksilver, and this medicine is proved to be effective. Also take 4 drachms each of the juice of iris and bull's gall, 2 drachms of suitable oil, mix all these together, put it in a pessary, give it to the woman, and this medicine will bring out all the decomposed matter of the womb. And it will deliver a woman of a dead child, and of her secundines, and it brings on menstruation. Again, give to the pregnant woman 2 drachms of asafetida 3 times daily, and let the stomach and back be anointed with oil and gall, and afterward let oil, ox gall, and asafetida be placed in the vulva with a feather.

[f. 219v] And the sicknesses that women have in childbearing come sometimes from the sickness of the child, and that may be because the child has grown considerably in his mother's womb before she has caught the dropsy; and this the midwife may well know, and the woman also. And sometimes the sickness comes through the frailty of the woman because she is not strong enough to deliver the child. And this may be in two ways: because of the great sickness that the woman has had and that has greatly weakened her; or because of the great anxiety of the woman, and if this is the first time that she has conceived for twelve years. Sometimes it comes from the blocking of the womb. And that may be due to two reasons: because fatness stops the mouth of the womb and holds back the blood that she should have been purged of before children were conceived; or sometimes it is because the child is dead in its mother's womb. And the signs are as follows: they feel no stirring or movement of the child inside; on the second day of labor the mouth smells evil; they feel much pain and distress about the navel; the face and the entire body waste away; they want things that are

contrarious to hem; anoþer is they haue moche wacche & litell
slepe; anoþer is þat þei hauen gret penaunce to make water & to
go to priuy, and also þat þei haue gret penaunce aboute þe
schare. And yf þe chyld comeþ nouʒt ouʒtwardes as he shulde,
the mydwif may helpen wel ynow withouten ony other medecynes, as I haue herafore tolde. But yf her greuaunce be of ony of
þese that I haue rehersed, make her a bath of hokkes [f. 220r], of
fenygrek, of lynsed, of wormode, of sothernewode & of par-
itorye, of fenell, & of mugwede soden in water, and lete bathe
hyr þerin a good whiles. And whan she comith oute of þe bath,
lete anoynt hir from þe navel dounward to þe priue membre with
butter & with deawte & with arragon, byfore & behynde hyr
also. And sithen make hir a fumigacion bynetheforth of spicenard ʒ i & *sem.* & of þe rotes of coste ʒ i. And also whanne she is
comen out of þe bath, yf she be a ryche woman, yeve hir ʒ i of
opibalsami with warme wyne; yf she be a pore woman, sethe þe
rotes of coste & of mugwede in wyne & do þerto ʒ ii of boles galle
& lete hir drynke it whan she comyth out of þe bath. Oþer tempre
borax ʒ ii with wyne & yeve hir that to drynke; oþer yeve hir the
jus of diptayn, ysope ana ʒ iii, argenti-vif ϑ *sem.*, & þis wyl casten
ouʒt þe childe quyk or dede & betir and yf it be yoven with a
trocisci of mirre after Rasis ordinaunce; take of mirre ʒ ii, lupinis ʒ
ii & *sem.*, of rue leves dried with wylde mynte, of puliol, id est,
woderofe, of sernum, of asefetida, serapium, opopanacium,
galbanum, gummi aromatici ana ʒ viii, of fyne maluesye as it
nedith. Make balles as it were table meyne of þe weight of ʒ ii,
eueryche of hem weying. Yeve her oone of hem with decoccion
of juniperii in wyne, for these ben good for hevy birthes & to
bringe forth þe secundines, & destroieth molam matricis. Yeff
these may not ben hadde, make a plastre of mugwede soden in
water & emplastre þe woman þerwith from þe navell to þe priue
membre, for it makith a woman sone be deliuered of hir child yf it
be quyk oþer dede in hir wombe & it drawith [f. 220v] oute þe
secundine. But lete it not ligge ful longe for it wyl drawe þe
moder out also. A noble, precious pouder* for women þat ben in
trauaylyng of child & for after throwes: take ʒ iii of þe scales of
cassiefistula & an ounce of saueray & another ounce of ysope;
poudre alle these in fere and yeve it þe woman with þe jus of
vervayne ywarmyd. And hit ydronke, it makith hyr sone to be

*MS. margin: *A special pouder.*

harmful to them; they wake a lot and sleep little; they have a great trouble in making water and going to the privy, and also they have great discomfort about the genitals. And if the child does not come out as it should, the midwife can help well enough without any other medicines, as I have previously described. But if her sickness be any of the ones that I have mentioned, make her a bath of mallows, [f. 220r] fenugreek, linseed, wormwood, southernwood, pellitory, fennel, and mugwort boiled in water, and let her bathe in it for a good time. And when she comes out of the bath, see that she is anointed from the navel downward to the privy member with butter, deute, and ointment of Aragon,* both in front and behind. And afterward make her a fumigation underneath of 1  ounces of spikenard and 1 ounce of roots of costmary. And also when she comes from the bath, if she is a rich woman, give her 1 ounce of the juice of the balsam tree in warm wine; if she is a poor woman, boil roots of costmary and artemisia in wine, add to it 2 ounces of bull's gall, and let her drink the mixture when she comes from the bath. Or mix 2 ounces of borax with wine and give her that to drink; or give her 3 drachms each of the juice of dittany, hyssop, half a scruple of mercury, and this medicament will cast out the child alive or dead, and even more successfully if it is given with a pill of myrrh, according to Rhazes' instruction; take 2 ounces of myrrh, 2½ ounces of lupins, 8 drachms each of rue leaves dried with wild mint, thyme, that is, woodruff, mountain willow, asafetida, orchis, juice of panax, galbanum, aromatic gum, and some good malmsey as required. Make pills like small tablets, each weighing 2 drachms. Give her one of them with an infusion of junipers in wine, for these are good for difficult births, to bring out the secundines and destroy the mola of the womb. If these cannot be obtained, make a plaster of artemisia boiled in water and plaster the woman with it from the navel to the privy member, for it makes a woman quickly give birth to a child, whether it is alive or dead in her womb, and it draws [f. 220v] out the secundine. But let it not remain there very long, for it will draw out the uterus also. A fine, valuable powder for women who are in labor and for pangs afterward: take 3 drachms of the pods of cassia fistula, an ounce of savory, and another ounce of hyssop; powder all these together and give it to the woman in the juice of vervain warmed. And this potion when drunk causes her to be quickly

* M.E.D. s.v. Aragon adj. cites vnguentum aragon as a medicament.

deliuered, and it drawith out þe secundine. Also it makith a woman þat is stopped sone to be deliuered by þe purgacion of hyr bloode. Also ciclamen ystrawed vnder a woman whiles she is trauayling it makith her sone to be deliuered.

The jus of vervayn doth also, ydronke. Oþer, lete hyr drynke an eyeschell full of þe jus of leek oþer of dyptayne, hokkes; also sauen, also a gret myght to deliueren a woman of childe. And so hath þe water of a mannes leer that he hath wasshen in his hondes. Tokens* whan a woman shall be deliuered of childe been gret sterynges & mevynges in hir wombe & oþerwhiles all þe wombe mevith vp to þe stomak and makith a woman to haue gret wylle to caste; & she hath moche hevinesse about þe navell & þan þe childe sterith faste to passen from his moder. Than lete stoppe hir nosethrilles þat þe spirites mowe go downe to þe moder and comforten hyr of hir birthen. And lete gyrden hyr with a gyrdell of an hertys skyn. And yef she swowne, lete putt swete smellyng thinges at hir nose, and lete froten the soles of hir fete & þe pawmes of hir handes with kene, bitynge thynges as with vynegre & salt. Baume, id est, opobalsami ymade in maner of a suppositorie makith [f. 221r] a woman ben deliuered of childe; and it drawith out þe secundine also but it makith hir bareyne euermor after. And þe jus of rue & of mugwede makith a woman sone be deliuered of childe though it be deede in hir wombe; & it is profitable to make hem to snese with pouder of peper & of castory & caste it in her nose. And þe jus of þe saturey ydronke makith a woman sone be deliuered of childe, & yf þe herbe be plasterd to her wombe, it makith þe childe come out quyk or dede. A precious stone, that highte Iaspis,†hathe a gret vertue to helpe women that they were deliuered of childe. Also, done yeven a woman þat hathe a dede childe in her wombe þe mylk of a becche medled with hony & make a plaster of wormote & bynde hit to hir left hype. Also womans mylk & oyle togeder ydronke makith a woman to be deliuered of childe. Also $R_x$: sauine, gladiolarum, id est yreos, abrotani, rute, diptani, isopi, saturei ana 3 *sem*., bene terantur cum vino optimo albo ʒ iii, & bibatur, & cito liberabitur.

*MS. margin: *Tokens*.
† Iaspis: MS. Isapis.

delivered, and it draws out the secundine. It also makes a woman who is stopped up to have her purgation straightaway. Also, cyclamen spread under a woman while she is in labor makes her give birth quickly.

The juice of vervain does the same thing when drunk. Alternatively, let her drink an eggshell full of the juice of leek or dittany, and mallows. These and savin also have great power to deliver a woman of her child. And the water from a man's skin that he has washed his hands in also has the same power. Signs that a woman is about to give birth are much stirring and movement in the womb, and sometimes all of the womb moves up to the stomach, causing the woman to have a great desire to give birth; and she feels very heavy about the navel, and the child bestirs itself vigorously to pass from its mother. Then have her nostrils stopped, so that the vital spirits can go down to the uterus, and encourage her with her burden. And have her put on a girdle of hart's skin. And if she faints, have sweet-smelling things placed at her nose, and rub the soles of her feet and the palms of her hands with sharp, biting things, such as vinegar and salt. Balm, that is, juice of the balsam tree made in the manner of a suppository, causes [f. 221r] a woman to be delivered of a child; it draws out the secundine also, but it causes her to be barren ever after. And the juice of rue and artemisia causes a woman quickly to be delivered of her child though it is dead in her womb. It is also helpful to make the patient sneeze with pepper powder and castory powder by throwing them up her nose. And a drink of savory juice causes a woman quickly to be delivered of her child, and if the herb is plastered on her womb it makes the child come out alive or dead. A precious stone called jasper has great power to help women in childbirth. Also, for a woman who has a dead child in her womb, give the juice of a beech tree mixed with honey, make a plaster of wormwood, and fasten it to her left hip. Woman's milk and oil drunk together make a woman give birth. Another prescription: half a drachm each of savin, gladiola, that is, iris, southernwood, rue, dittany, hyssop, savory; let them be well crushed in 3 ounces of the best white wine and drunk, and she will be quickly delivered.

*De mola matricis.*

Mola matricis is in two maners: oon maner is mola whan it is a wikked nature & þan it is a flesshy lumpe the whiche a litel & a litel encrecith & wexith in the marice, as it were in liknesse of a childe verilich conceyved. In þe whiche is enchesounde & caused as þe moder vnderstondith of þe womans owne seed moche withholden in þe marice with lakking of mannes doyng. For if it were of a mannes seed þat it were not myghty that it shulde haue lyf thorough reson of þe whiche thyng þe vertu naturall & þe hete naturall of þe marice, þey maken [f. 221v] there a flesshy lumpe without lyf. Anoþer is cleped mola nouȝt trewe, and þat is in two maners. Oone is þat is engendred of wynde a litell & a litell gadred in þe marice enchesonyng þerin gret wyndynesse. The signe of it is yf þe marice be touched, it makith a sowne as it were in a tympanyst, id est, in soche an ydropesie þat is engendred & ygadred þorough* wynd. Anoþer maner is mola þat is nought verrye. The whiche is engendred þorugh foule roten humours & grete & tough to dissoluen in þe marice. And þer tho foule gret humours maken gret swellyng as it were anoþer maner of ydropesie þat is cleped Alchites. And þese two maners of molis is all oon cure. And, also I haue seyd, mola wexith in þe marice as it were a child quyk & mevith but not so swyftelye. But it mevith dedely & seldome & it castith out wynde oþerwhiles fro þe marice & oþerwhiles lumpes off flesshe.
*Cure* of þis maladie is riȝt hard & longe or it be do. Fyrst make hyr a bath of herbes into þe whiche þe woman shall wende. Fyrst to soften hyr bones & hyr joyntes: Take all þe malewes, fenygrek herbe, baume, primerolle, lilies, camomill, wormode, calamynte, sothernewode, pollipodii branche, vrsyne, violet, paritorie, fenell leves, & lynsed, & make herof a stuphe & whan þe woman hath sete heryn longe ynough than in her comyng out, yeve hir two dramys of this trocisci Rasis with þe jus of rue & of nept & anoynte her navell douneward dialtea, olio liliorum, may butter þat is fresshe & do wrappe all her bodie all aboute with an hoot dowble schete; than make hyr a fumigacion of spycenard & of comyn and of costi. Whan þat ys [f. 222r] done, lete anoynte hir previte withinforth thus. Take bolys galle ℥ vi, oyle ℥ ii, medle hem togeders and make an oynement & do þerto ℥ i euforbii, the

*þorough: MS. þorouhg.

*Concerning the mola of the womb.*

Mola of the womb is of two kinds: one kind is virulent in nature, a fleshy lump which increases and grows little by little in the womb, having all the appearance of a child properly conceived. This kind of mola occurs when the uterus accepts the woman's own seed [ovum] kept back unfertilized in the womb. For if it comes from a man's seed that is not powerful enough to be viable as a result of natural virtue and natural heat of the womb, in consequence, [f. 221v] a lifeless, fleshy lump is produced. The other kind is called a false mola, and this is of two kinds. One is the result of wind gathering little by little in the womb and causing great windiness inside. The indication of it is if the womb is touched, it makes a sound as if it were in a tympanites,* that is, in the kind of dropsy which is produced and fostered through wind. The false mola can be another kind. It springs from evil decaying humors, large and difficult to dissolve in the womb. And those large, evil humors make a great swelling there, like a different kind of dropsy that is called ascites. And there is one cure for these two kinds of mola. And, as I have also said, the mola grows in the womb as though it were a child, alive and moving, though not so swiftly. But it moves without life and infrequently, and sometimes it casts wind out of the womb, sometimes lumps of flesh.

The cure for this malady is very difficult and takes a long time before it is effective. First, make her a bath of herbs for the woman to go into. First, to soften her bones and joints: take all the mallows, the herb fenugreek, balm, primrose, lilies, camomile, wormwood, calamint, southernwood, frond of polypody, garlic, violet, pellitory, fennel leaves, and linseed, and make a bath of them; and when the woman has remained in it long enough, as she comes out give her 2 drachms of Rhazes pills with the juice of rue and catmint, and anoint her navel downward with a preparation from marshmallows, oil of lilies, fresh May butter, and wrap a hot double sheet over her entire body; then make a fumigation for her of spikenard, cumin, and costmary. When that is [f. 222r] done, have her privity anointed inside thus: take 6 drachms of bull's gall, 2 drachms of oil, mix them together, make an ointment, and add to it 1 ounce of milkwort,

* A form of dropsy in which the body, if thumped, sounds like a drum.

jus of savyne ℥ ii, peleter of spayne ℥ i, scamonie ℥ iiii, rotes of diptayne ℥ i; make pouder of all þese, put it in þe boles galle & medle hem togedres well & with a longe fether anoynt her withyn also depe as þou may & putt yn ynough & lete hyr ligge so hir hede lowe & hir taylende high. And yf she worthe owher yholpen þis wyl shewe sume doyng. For þis medecyne will deliuere, þough þer were a childe quyk or dede. Anoþer maner of trocisci be these: R$_x$: asefetide ℈ x, & grana xvi, gumi armoniaci, galbani, serapii, opopanaci, agarici, foliorum cene, lupini, castorei, olei benedicti ana ℈ ii & *sem.*, boracis ℥ ii, bidellii ℈ i, baccarum lauri, pionearum, pollipodii nuchi, ceresorum, seminis petrosilii, juniperii, feni, arostologie rotundae & longae, xilobalsami, carpobalsami, cassie lignii, ciperii, genciane, centaurie, rute, macis, cucube, savine, jus achory, asari, nepite, calamenti, diptani, reubarbi, nardi, squinanti, origani, croci, carui, anisi, rubie, mororum ana granorum 25, suca rute, mellis, vini aromatici, ana quartern i; coquantur, id est, sethe þe jus of rue, þe wyne of hony a litell, þanne ley asa, gummi armoniaci, galbanum, serapium, & borarum, & ley all these infuse a nyght & a day; on þe morewe sethe hem ayen & þan clense hem þorough a clothe. And sethe þat is so clensed till þe jus of þat rue & þe wyne be consumed; than all þe spices & þe gummes ypoudred and so put þerto & make of þe weigt of ℈ ii euerych, yif oon balle in mola as I sayd before. And also make a suppositorie of ℈ i of þese balles: farine, stafizacrie, of euforbie, of pileter of spayne, scamonie ana ℈ i, bolis gallis ℈ i, make a litell bagge of [f. 222v] lynnen cloth þat is well ouerwered & make a suppositorie, for it will brynge forth bothe dede child, yf ony there be, & it bringith forth þe secundine & þe blode, and it bringith forth lumpes of þe mola. But yet yeve hyr to drynke a balle with þe jus of diptayne, of saueray ana ℈ ii, quyksiluer ℈ *sem.*; this is oon of þe best yf a woman trauaile of childe & it be dede, to deliuer her þerof. Also anoþer pissorie is: take jus of wormode, of mugwede, of puliole, of diptani, or origani, of saueray, of savine ana ℈ ii, of boles galle ℈ xxxii, of pileter, of gladon, of lauriall, of oyle, of clene hony, ana ℥ *sem.*; medle all these togeders & with an instrument caste it into

2 ounces of the juice of savin, 1 ounce of pellitory of Spain, 4 ounces of scammony, 1 ounce of roots of dittany; make a powder of all these, put it in the bull's gall, mix them well together, and with a long feather anoint the place within as deeply as you can and put in enough, and let her lie so that her head is low and her bottom high. And if she can be helped in any way, this will show in the result, for this medicine will make her deliver even though there were a child alive or dead. Pills of a different kind are as follows: take 10 drachms and 16 grains of asafetida, 2½ drachms each of gum ammoniac, galbanum, orchis, juice of panax herb, agaric, leaves of chive, lupins, castory, oil benedicta, 2 ounces of borax, 1 drachm of vine-palm, 25 grains each of laurel berries, peonies, seed of polypody, honeycomb, seeds of rock parsley, juniper, fennel, the round and the long birthwort, balsam wood, shrub balsam, wood of cassia, galingale, gentian, centaury, rue, mace, cucumber, savin, juice of acorus,* hazelwort, catmint, calamint, dittany, rhubarb, spikenard, camel's hay, origanum, saffron, caraway, anise, madder, mulberries, 1 measure each of the juice of rue, honey, aromatic vines; let them be cooked, that is, boil the juice of rue, wine, and honey a little, and then put in mastic, Armenian bole, galbanum, orchis, and borax, and infuse all these for a day and a night; boil them again the next day and strain them through a cloth. And boil the part that is strained until the juice of the rue and the wine is consumed; then add all the spices and gums powdered and make everything the weight of 2 drachms and give one pill, in the case of the mola previously described. And also make a suppository of 1 drachm of these pills: 1 drachm each of flour, stavesacre, milkwort, pellitory of Spain, scammony, and bull's gall, make a little bag of [f. 222v] linen cloth that is threadbare and prepare a suppository, for it will bring out the dead child if there is one, the secundine, the blood, and lumps of the mola. Give her a pill to drink with 2 drachms each of the juice of dittany, and savory, half a scruple of quicksilver; this is one of the best means of delivering a woman who is in labor and the child is dead. Another pessary is: take 2 drachms each of juice of wormwood, artemisia, wild thyme, dittany, origanum, savory, and savin, 32 drachms of bull's gall, half an ounce each of pellitory, iris, laurel, oil, clear honey; mix all these together, and with an instrument put

---

* Aromatic plant sometimes identified with calamus.

her wombe by þe priue membre with a litell pouder of euforbie &
a litell of ellebori albi* ana ʒ ii. For þis pissorie destroieth all
maner molis of þe marice & bringith forth with gret violence.
And þough a woman were stopped foure yere or fyve, it wyll
doon his dever *hoc Augustinus*. But fyrst, whan þe woman is
comen out of þe bath aforesaid, first after þat she is anoynted &
þan wrapped in a shete & þe balles aforesaid, þou shalt make her
to snese; & whan sche is þus yserved, þou shalt tene hir & make
her angerd† & þan þou shalt make hyr aferd & whan thou haste
þus ydoone, þou shalt yeve hyr þe pissaries aforesaid or þe
suppositorie. Also, in mola matricis: ther was a woman & she
was deliuered by þe wyndyng of two towailes aboute hir
myddell & twoo stikkis; the oon was bounden on þe oone syde
off þe woman & þe other wounde on þe other syde of hyr till þe
wombe of hyr was made right small, & þe woman hadde riȝt
fayre children yit þerafter. Or els, yeve hyr trocisci of myrre þa[t]
Rasis makith [f. 223r] in his boke of Almosorum þe whiche ben
these: take mirre ʒ iii, lupinis ʒ v, leves of drie rue, of wylde
mynte, of woderove, madir, ameos, asafetida, serapium, apo-
ponak, galbani, gummi armoniaci ana ʒ ii; make a trocisci with
good wyne aromatici;‡ yeve ʒ ii of hem with decoccion of
duretik§ sedes & of savyne, madir, and of saueray ana ʒ ii.

*The 11 Chapiter is of þe Secundine that is withholden yn women after
chyld beryng.*

Secundine is a litell skynne þat goth abowte þe childe whiles
he is in his moder wombe, right as þer is an inner skynne that
goth abowte a nutte kernell. And oþerwhiles a woman is deliuered of þat secundine whan she is deliuered of hir child; and
oþerwhiles she is deliuered of hir child & þe secundine levith
stille behynde withyn her for þe gret feblenes of hir marice; & þat
may come of moche fastyng, oþer of gret angre, wrathe, oþer
smytyng, oþer summe longe fluxe of þe wombe, þe whiche
thinges sleth a chyld in his moder wombe. But þanne þe moder
deliueryth hyr of þe chyld but þe secundine levith still withyn þe
moder

*Ellebori albi has been inserted in a sixteenth-century hand.
† angerd: MS. an angerd.
‡ aromatici: MS. romanici.
§ duretik: MS. duretif.

the pessary in her womb via the privy member, with a little powder of milkwort and a little of white hellebore, 2 drachms of each. For this pessary destroys all kinds of mola of the womb and expels with great force. And although a woman be stopped up for four or five years, it will be effective according to Augustine. But first, when the woman comes out of the bath already described, as soon as she is oiled, wrapped in a sheet, and [given] the pills previously mentioned, cause her to sneeze, and when she does so, make her distressed, angry, and then frightened, and when you have done so, give her the pessaries previously mentioned or the suppository. Also, in the case of the mola of the womb; there was a woman, and she was freed of it by winding two towels about her middle and using two sticks; one stick was bound on the one side of her and the other twisted on the other side until her stomach was squeezed very small, and the woman still had very beautiful children afterward. Alternatively, give her pills of myrrh devised by Rhazes [f. 223r] in his book of Almansor, which are these: take 3 ounces of myrrh, 5 drachms of lupins, 2 drachms each of leaves of dried rue, wild mint, woodruff, madder, bishop's-weed, asafetida, orchis, opopanax, galbanum, gum ammoniac; make pills with good aromatic wine; give 2 drachms of them in an infusion of 2 drachms each of diuretic seeds, savin, madder, and savory.

*The eleventh chapter is concerned with the secundine that is retained in women after childbirth.*

Secundine is a little skin that goes about the child while he is in his mother's womb, just as there is an inner skin that goes around the nut kernel. And sometimes a woman is delivered of that secundine when she gives birth to her child, and sometimes she gives birth to her child and the secundine remains behind inside her because of the great weakness of her womb; and that may be the result of much fasting, great anger, wrath, beating, or some prolonged flux of the womb, which things kill the child in his mother's womb. And then the mother gives birth to the child, but the secundine remains within her.

And þe mydwif shuld anoynt her hondes & with hir nayles
pullen owte þe secundine yf she mowe; & yf she mowe not, bore
holes in a stole and lette hyr sytte þeron, and make a fumigacion
vndernethe of þe hornes of gete & of hir clawes of her fete so þat
þe smoke smyʒt vpright to her priue membre. Or els, take salt
oþer asshen of anyse* ybrent & tempre hem with water & yeve
her to drynke. Also make a bathe of wormode & of hokkis and
holyhokkis, calamynte, fenigreke, origani, & make her sitten in
þat bath vp to þe navell. And whan she comyth out of þat bath,
anoynte hyr from þe navell dounward [f. 223v] with fressh butter
& with oyle de bay and arragon & with dewte & with the same
anoynt her sides and her bak aboute her reynes. Also, take þe jus
of parcili & of leke & medle hem with [oyle] of puliole & yeve
hem to drynk oþer þe jus of barage. And þat will drawe out þe
secundine. Et sic require in sufficacione menstruorum.

*The 12 Chapiter is to make a woman able to conceyven chyld yf God wyll.*

Fyrst, yf she be repleted of hyr menstruys, do clense hyr with
medecines in retencione menstruorum & in suffocacione menstruorum, with bathes & stuphes. Oþer take calamynt, nept,
fenell, paritorie, saueray, Isop, mugwede, rue, wormode, anise,
comyn, rosemaryn, thim, puliol† riall, & mountayn origanum
ana *m.* i, wyne a galon, water six galons and sethe hem or yeve
hyr to ete þis medecyne. Take pouder of clowes iii vnces, foure
yelkis of rawe eyren & medle þe pouder & þe yelkis togeders and
bake it on an hote stone and yeve hit the woman fastyng foure
dayes withouten drynke a good whyle after it is eten. Also, for
man or for woman make an emplastre of iiii yelkis of rawe eyren,
of pouder of clowes ℥ *sem.*, of saffron ℈ i. And first anoynte with
hote oyle of roses on þe mouthe of the stomak & strewe þeron
summe of þe pouder and make an emplastre and ley hit to.

*The 13 Chapiter is of bledyng ouermoche after that sche hath hadde her
chylde.*

The women þat bleden oþerwhiles to moche after þat þei haue
bore her children, and þat makith hem full feble. But þou ne shalt
nought in this caas yeven hyr [f. 224r] no medecines þat ben

*anyse: MS. anyne.
† puliol: MS. pilule.

The midwife should anoint her hands and with her nails pull out the secundine if she can; and if she cannot, bore holes in a stool and let the woman sit on it, and make underneath a fumigation from goats' horns and the claws of their feet, so that the smoke strikes right up to her privy member. Alternatively, take salt or ashes of burnt anise and mix them with water and give them her to drink. Also make a bath of wormwood, mallows, hollyhocks, calamint, fenugreek, origanum, and make her sit in that bath up to the navel. And when she comes out of that bath, anoint her from the navel downward [f. 223v] with fresh butter, oil of bay, Aragon, and deute and with the same preparation anoint her sides and back around her kidneys. Also, take the juice of parsley and leek, mix them with wild thyme oil and give them to her to drink, or the juice of borage. And that will draw out the secundine. And do the same for stoppage of menstruation.

*The twelfth chapter is on how to make a woman conceive a child if God wills.*

First, if she is full of menstrual blood, have her cleansed with medicines for the retention and suppression of menstruation, with baths and immersions. Alternatively, take 1 handful each of calamint, catmint, fennel, pellitory, savory, hyssop, artemisia, rue, wormwood, anise, cumin, rosemary, thyme, pennyroyal, and mountain origanum, a gallon of wine, 6 gallons of water, boil them, and have her take this medicine. Take 3 ounces of powder of cloves and 4 yolks of raw eggs, mix the powder and the yolks together, bake on a hot stone, and give to the woman after a four-day fast, and make her abstain from fluids for some time afterwards. Also, for either a man or woman, make a plaster of 4 yolks of raw eggs, half an ounce of powder of cloves, 1 drachm of saffron. First anoint with hot oil of roses on the orifice of the stomach, spread on it some of the powder, make a plaster, and lay it on it.

*The thirteenth chapter is concerned with excessive bleeding after childbirth.*

Women sometimes bleed too much after childbirth, and this makes them very weak. But you should not in this case [f. 224r] give her any medicines that are

comfortatiue* nor bathes noþer stronge striktories but oþer
medecines, as it was tolde before in þe chapiter of to moche
flowyng of blode. Lete hyr blode vnder þe ancle on the oon† fote;
and another day vnder þe toþer ancle. And yeve hyr þanne oþer
medecyns as it was saide herebefore as we shuld haue yeve hyr
medecyns that were tolde in þe chapiter of withholdyng of blode.
And sume women haue corrupte mater as quyttour passyng away
from hem. And oþerwhiles suche mater passith from hem in stede
of blode; and oþerwhiles with þe blodes that þe blode þei shuld be
purged of. And yf þey be olde women oþer women þat be bareyn,
it nedith noȝt to yeve hem no medecyns þerof; yf they be yonge
women, lete sethe kerslokkis oþer tormentill & fyve leves grasse
oþer skyrwittes in wyne. And lete hyr sitten ouer þe smoke þerof
þat it may come to hyre pryue membre.
Oþer, take puliole & make a pouder þerof & putte it into a bagge
so brode & so longe that it will ouer hille bothe priue membres of
þe woman. And all warme ley it to thilke membres & bynde it
faste þat it falle noȝt away.

  Wowndes of þe marice ben yheled with þe jus of plantayne &
of solatri, and with þe whyte of an egge & þe jus of purcelane ana
ʒ vi, gummi dragaganti, gummi arabici ana ʒ vi. Infundantur &
it wyl be lyche a muscillage worthy and good to kele & to hele.
And yf þy vynes‡ be broke they schull be heled with þe jus of
centorie & with bole & with sangdragon & with the sedes of
mirtellis and with þe rounde aristologum, and [f. 224v] with
suche oþer medecyns. Also, take this for a principall medecyn
for all maner woundes in þis place, yf it come of moche hete, as
comenly it dothe, more þan of colde. Take of gum arabici & gum
dragaganti white ʒ vi, & enfuse it in two ounces of water of roses
& a ounce of oyle of mirtilles with pouder of mastyk & olibani ana
Ɔ vi. And all these schull be made in oone confeccion as in
manere of an oynement. And lete a priue woman ley þer þe sore
is this medecyn afornsaid, noght oonly to woundes of this place
but also in all oþer places & to chynes, clyftes in þe lippes and of
þe mowthe. Another medecyn for þat same: take gum arabie,
dragagante ʒ iiii, borace ʒ ii, camphore, bole, alcanne,
sangdraconis ana ʒ i, masticis, mirtilles, ceruse, olibani, litargiri

*comfortatiue: MS. corfortatiue.
†oon: MS. too.
‡vynes: MS. wynes.

comforting, nor baths nor strong medicated compresses, but
other medicines such as were described earlier in the chapter on
hemorrhage. Have her bled under the ankle of one foot, and
another day under the other ankle. Then give her other
medicines as before stated here that we should give, such
medicines as were described in the chapter on the retention of
blood. And some women have decaying matter when they have
a discharge, and sometimes such matter passes from them
instead of blood; and sometimes bleeding comes with the blood
that they should be purged of. And if they are old women or
women that are barren, there is no need to give them medicines.
If they are young women, boil watercress, septfoil, cinquefoil,
or water parsnips in wine. And let her sit over the smoke of
them so that it reaches her privy member.

Alternatively, take wild thyme, make a powder of it, and put
it in a bag of sufficient breadth and length to cover both privy
members of the woman. And put it on hot and fasten it securely
so that it cannot fall off.

Sores of the womb are healed with the juice of plantain and
morel, and 6 ounces each of white of egg, juice of purslane, gum
tragacanth, and gum arabic. Let this medication be given, and it
will act like an excellent mucilage, good for cooling and healing.
And if the veins are broken, they should be healed with juice of
centaury, Armenian bole, sandragon, myrtle seeds, round
birthwort, and [f. 224v] with other similar medicines. Also, take
this as the main medicine for all kinds of sores in this place if
they are due to excessive heat, as they usually are, rather than
due to cold. Take 6 drachms each of gum arabic and white gum
tragacanth, and steep the mixture in 2 ounces of water of roses,
an ounce of myrtle oil, and 6 scruples each of powder of mastic
and olibanum. And all these should be made into one
preparation like an ointment. And let a discreet woman apply
this medication where the sore is, not only to inflammation in
this place but to all other places, lacerations, cracks in the lips,
and the mouth. Another medicine for the same thing: take gum
arabic, 4 drachms of gum tragacanth, 2 drachms of borax, 1
drachm each of camphor, Armenian bole, alkannet,* sandragon,
half a drachm each of mastic, myrtle, white lead, olibanum,
litharge,

* See *M.E.D.* s.v. alkanne (t n. The plant or its root was used as a styptic or
coloring.

ana ʒ *sem.*, olei bodegari ʒ iiii, aqua rosarum ʒ viii; lay ʒe gum dragani & þe borace in þe rose water, infuse a day & a nyght tyll þei be all relented; thanne cole hem thorough a shyre clothe till þei be brouʒt all clene thorough; than alle þe toþer spices made into sotill pouder & ymedled with þe oyle afornseyd & with this muscillage tyl þey be riʒt well incorporate & put to vse whan it nedith. This medecyn is good for all maner cancres, cancrettis, hote woundes, horisipilatus, id est, wyldefiris, felons, carbuncles, mormalis of colre adust & all suche other. Yf þe woundes come þorgh colde, take þe muscillage of fenigreke ʒ iiii, of sarcocoll, infuse in decoccion of camomille, spicenard, masticis, mirre, cinamoni, castorei ana Ɖ i, right subtylly made into pouder; medle hem togeder with womans mylk & with þe jus of planteyn ana ʒ ii & *sem.*; when they ben well ymedled, do it to þe maladie in þe priue membre for this medecyne fordothe all þe [f. 225r] maladies of þat place yf it be curable with medecyns.

*De cancris & vlceribus matricis.*

Cancryng and festres of þe marice comyn of olde woundes of þe marice þat wer noʒt well heled, but þat maner of syknesse we wyl speke but litell of for phisiciens sayne þat cancres þat ben hydde it is better þat þei be vncured than cured or heled. But natheles, this oynement is good þerfore & for ʒicching also & blaynes þat ben in þe moder. Take a gourde þat is rype & pare hym withouten & clense hym also of þat that is withyn hym & after þat stampe hym riʒt small & þan sett it in a potte on þe fyre with oyle of roses, & wex, & shepes talewe, & when þey be well soden, caste þerto pouder of mastik & of olibanum, & lete hem boyle wel togeder. And sithen þorough a clothe, clense & þerwith anoynt hem withynforth. And þis oþer oynement is good also for brennyng & for scaldyng; but whan suche a sore is anoynted þerwith ley þer above Ivy leves soden in wyne. A sowdyng medecyn for alle maner cancres maters; take þis medecyne for all. Fyrste take rotes of rede dokkis *li. sem*, rotes of yris *li.* i, sethe these rotes in clere water thre quartes, and a quart of whyt wyne; sethe hem till a

4 ounces of oil from the store, 8 drachms of water of roses. Put the gum tragacanth and the borax in the rose water, steep a day and a night until they are all dissolved; then strain them through a light cloth until they come through entirely clean; and have all the other spices made into a fine powder and mixed with the previously mentioned oil, as well as with this mucilage, until they are entirely blended, and then put to use when necessary. This medicine is good for all kinds of cancers, tumors, hot sores, erysipelas, that is, wildfire, sores, carbuncles, ulcers from a morbid secondary form of black bile, and all other such complaints. If the sores are the result of cold, take 4 drachms of mucilage of fenugreek, sarcocolla* infused in a mixture of 1 scruple each of camomile, spikenard, mastic, myrrh, cinnamon, and castory, skillfully made into a powder. Mix them all together with 2½ drachms of woman's milk and juice of plantain; when they are well mixed, apply it to the disorder in the privy member because this medicine does away with all [f. 225r] the maladies of that place if they can be cured by medicines.

*Concerning cancers and ulcers of the womb.*

Cancers and festerings of the womb come from old injuries of the womb that have not healed well, but that kind of sickness we will hardly mention because doctors say that, with regard to hidden cancers, it is better that they should be uncured rather than cured or treated. Nevertheless, this ointment is good for such things and for itching and blisters in the uterus. Take a ripe gourd,† pare it and clean it inside, grind it very small, and put in a pot on the fire with oil of roses, wax, sheep's tallow, and when they are well boiled, throw in mastic powder and olibanum, and let them boil well together. And afterward strain through a cloth and anoint patients with the medicament inside. And this ointment is also good for burning and scalding; after using it on a sore, place ivy leaves boiled in wine on top. A strengthening medicine for all kinds of cancerous complaints; take this medicine for them all. First take half a pound of roots of red dock,‡ 1 pound of roots of iris, boil these roots in 3 quarts of clear water and a quart of white wine; boil them down to half a

---

* A Persian gum.
† Probably a cucumber is meant.
‡ *Rumex sanguineus*: a coarse, weedy herb often used in medicine. The common dock was (and still is) a popular antidote for nettle stings.

potell. And put þerto a litell hony, as ʒ vi with þe whyte of eyren xvi, and clarifie it & wasshe þe priue membre þerwith riʒt well; þan take coton right wel ytosed & put þat coton esely into a lynnen poket; than wete þat poket with þat coton, and esely it shall be clensed, and do away þe filthe þerfrom. Than make this enplaster: take gume dragaganti albi, gume of arabie ana ʒ ii, ley hem infuse in water of roses till þey be riʒt softe [f. 225v]; than take also of aloes, wasshe of ceruse, ywasshe of frankencense, of sandragon ana ʒ ii, of litarge, of gold ʒ i, wex ʒ ii, of oyle of roses ʒ vi; make a brasen morter riʒt hote & putt þerto þe wex & with þe muscillage of draganti and of þe gum of arabie & medle hem right well & lete hem sumdele kele; þan put in þe oyle of roses with þe poudres, and medle hem right wel togedres. And whan they be right well encorporate and is right colde, putte þerto campher with a litell more oyle of roses ygrounde. And hereof make prove medecynes, for it is right good.

*For swelling of womennes legges whan þei be with chylde.*

**W**omen whan they ben with childe hir legges wyll swelle. Than take þat þat lyeth in þe smethys trowgh vnder his gryndyng stone & drie it and make pouder of hit and medle hit with vynegre, and anoynte þerwith þat place þat swellith so. Other, ley it þeron in maner of a plaster. Oþer take þe floure of benen mele & medle hit with vynegre & with oyle and lay hit or þerof on þe swellyng. Or els, anoynt hit with blak sope, and sithen lay a plaster þeron of eldren leves fryed by hymsylf in a panne withouten ony other liquor. And þe same medecyns ben good for swellyng of a mannes fete oþer legges þat jorneyeth by the weyes.

*Ad menstrua prouocanda*: R$_x$: parsily rotes, fenell ana *m.* i, of isop leves, saueray, betonice, foliorum lauri, rosmarin, lauendre ana *m. sem.*, nepte *m.* iii, dyptani, rute, arthemisie ana ʒ ii & *sem.*, carui, pollipodi ʒ iiii, vini albi lagenam i, tonsis & coctis ad medietatem & collatis & iterum coctis cum croco Ɵ i, gariofoli ʒ [f. 226r] ii, granorum paradisi ʒ *sem.*, mellis* ʒ vi, sillicie fetide. R$_x$: turbitti albi granosi, colloquintida cusentem aloe, citrini, zinziberi, epithemi ana Ɵ ii, sone ʒ ii, ellibori albi & nigri, croci, piretri, seminis cicute, seminis anisi, ameos, carui, sinapii & nasturcii ana Ɵ *sem.*, reubarbii *sem.*, apii, galbani, opoponacis,

*mellis: MS. molla.

gallon. And add a little honey, say, 6 drachms with the whites of 16 eggs, clarify the mixture, and wash the privy member carefully with it; then take well-combed cotton and put the cotton gently into a linen bag; then wet the bag with the cotton, and it will clean the cancer without difficulty, and take away the dirt from it. Then make this plaster: take 2 drachms each of gum of white tragacanth and gum arabic, put them to steep in water of roses until they are very soft; [f. 225v] then take also 2 drachms each of aloes, lotion of white lead, lotion of frankincense, sandragon, 1 drachm of litharge of gold, 2 drachms of wax, 6 drachms of oil of roses; make very hot a brass mortar and put in it the wax, the oil of tragacanth, and the gum arabic, mix them well together, and let them cool slightly; then put in the oil of roses with the powders and mix them thoroughly. And when they are well blended and very cold, add camphor with a little more of the oil of crushed roses. And from this mixture make tested medical potions, for it is very good.

*For swelling of women's legs when they are pregnant.*

The legs of pregnant women will swell. Then take what lies in the smithy's trough beneath his grinding stone, dry it, make a powder of it, mix it with vinegar, and anoint the place that swells with it. Alternatively, lay it on like a plaster. Or take bean-meal flour, mix it with vinegar and oil, and put it on the swelling. Or else anoint it with black soap, and afterward lay a plaster on it of elder leaves fried by themselves in a pan without any other liquor. And the same medicines are good for swelling in a man's feet or for legs that travel by the roads.

*To provoke menstruation*: Take 1 handful each of parsley roots, fennel, half a handful each of hyssop leaves, savory, betony, laurel leaves, rosemary, lavender, 3 handfuls of catmint, 2½ drachms of dittany, rue, artemisia, 4 drachms each of caraway, polypody, and a flagon of white wine; [have the herbs] cut, cooked thoroughly, strained and again cooked with 1 scruple of saffron, 2 ounces of cloves, [f. 226r] half a drachm of grains of paradise, 6 drachms of honey, fetid salt. Take 2 scruples each of white grains of terebinth, colocynth, pounded aloe, citron, ginger, thyme, 2 drachms of hemlock, half a scruple each of black and white hellebore, saffron, pellitory, hemlock seeds, anise seeds, bishop's-weed, caraway, mustard and nasturtium seed and rhubarb, 2½ drachms of parsley, galbanum, panax,

bidellii, asefetide ana ʒ ii & *sem.*, mirre elice olei benedicti ana ʒ ii, sarcocolle, castorei, diagredii, euforbii, esule, ligni aloes, centaurie, sticados ana Э i, agarici Э ii; fiant pillule cum succo porri dosis ʒ ii & *sem.*, cum decoccione supradicta.

*Emplastrum*: R$_x$: malbarum *m.* ii, millifolii, feniculi, ebuli, ana *m.* i, foliorum porri *m.* iii; scindantur minutissime & terantur & frixantur cum pauca aqua & fiat emplastrum circum circa totum ventrem vsque ad vuluam.

*Fomentacio*: R$_x$: radices iris quartern i, anisi ʒ i, rosimarini, calamenti, isopi, saturei, origani ana ʒ i; & coquantur tam in vino quam* in aqua & ponantur herbe in sacculo & post fomentacionem ponatur saculus ad vuluam ad molam matricis & ad fetum mortuum. R$_x$: seminis porri, apii, mirre, spicenardi, calaminis, squinanti, corticis cassiefistule ana ʒ ii; anisi fiat puluis & recipiatur mane non exitu a balneo, cum aqua, vino, melle, decoctionis saturie, isopi, diptani, rubie, inula,† nepite, iris, salsequii, abrotani, ana *m.* i. Item secundum Rasim: R$_x$: ase, aristologie rotunde & longe ana ʒ vi, mirre, agarici, nardi ana ʒ iii, fiant trocisci ponderis vnius‡ ʒ iii, cum decoccione juniperii, et sunt forte educentes embrionem. R$_x$: achori, asari, amomi, semina triplicis maratri ani ʒ i & grana§ xviii, anisi ʒ ii, aristologie longe,** arthemisie, cassieligni ana ʒ ii, Э ii, & grana ii, centauria minor ʒ i Э i, & granum i, centaurie maioris ʒ ii, dauci cretici ʒ ii, ellebori nigri ʒ i, folii lauri ʒ i & *sem.*, grana ix, liquerice ʒ iiii, lupinorum ʒ i, melancii ʒ ii, mirre ʒ vi Э ii, & grana iii, cirobi ʒ iii, stipteree ʒ vi, mace-[f. 226v] donici piretri ʒ ii Э ii, grana ii, piperis nigri ʒ v Э i, grana ii, ciperi ʒ i, seminis rute ʒ ii Э ii, grana ii, spicenardi ʒ ii & grana ii, sinicinis, id est classa, ʒ ii, squinanti ʒ i Э ii, & grana ii, apii, sauine ʒ i, xilobalsami ʒ i Э ii, & grana ii,

---

*quam: MS. quanto.
† inula: MS. ina.
‡ vnius: MS. vnus.
§ grana: MS. granci.
**longe: MS. longi.

vine-palm, and asafetida, 2 drachms each of myrrh, and drawn oil benedicta, 1 scruple each of gum arabic, castory, scammony, euphorbia, spurge, wood aloes, centaury, and French lavender, 2 scruples of larch fungus; let pills be made with leek juice in portions of 2½ drachms with the above-described mixture.

*A plaster*: Take 2 handfuls of mallows, 1 handful each of milfoil, fennel, and dwarf elder, 3 handfuls each of leaves of leeks; let them be cut very minutely, ground, and roasted with a little water, and let a circular plaster be put around the whole of the stomach up to the vulva.

*Fermentation*: Take 1 measure of roots of iris, 1 ounce of anise, 1 drachm each of rosemary, calamint, hyssop, savory, and origanum; let them be cooked in equal amounts of wine and water, and let the herbs be placed in a bag, and after fermentation let the bag be placed on the vulva for a mola of the womb and for a dead fetus. Take 2 drachms each of leek seeds, wild celery, myrrh, spikenard, calamint, camel's hay, and the rind of cassia fistula; have anise ground to powder, and let her take it early before having a bath, with water, wine, honey, and a decoction of 1 handful each of savory, hyssop, dittany, madder, elecampane, catmint, iris, dry salt, and southernwood. In like manner, according to Rhazes, take 6 drachms each of hazelwort, round and long birthwort, 3 drachms each of myrrh, larch fungus, and spikenard; have pills made, each 3 drachms in weight, with a potion of junipers, and they greatly assist in bringing forth the embryo. Take 1 drachm and 18 grains each of iris, hazelwort, tree nightshade, and seeds of three-leaf fennel, 2 drachms of anise, 2 drachms, 2 scruples, and 2 grains each of long birthwort, artemisia, and wood of cassia, 1 drachm, 1 scruple, and 1 grain of lesser centaury, 2 drachms of greater centaury, 2 drachms of carrots, 1 ounce of black hellebore, 1 drachms and 9 grains of laurel leaves, 4 drachms of licorice, 1 ounce of lupins, 2 drachms of fennel, 6 drachms, 2 scruples, and 3 grains of myrrh, 3 drachms of carob, 6 drachms of styptic, 2 drachms, 2 scruples, and 2 grains of Macedonian [f. 226v] pellitory, 5 drachms, 1 scruple, and 2 grains of black pepper, 1 drachm of galingale, 2 drachms, 2 scruples, and 2 grains of laurel seed, 2 drachms and 2 grains of spikenard, 2 drachms of potash, that is, gunpowder, 1 drachm, 2 scruples, and 2 grains of camel's hay, some parsley, 1 drachm of savin, 1 drachm, 2 scruples, and 2 grains of balsam wood,

pulegii, pionearum mundatarum ℨ ii & Ə i, gariofoli ℨ ii, radicis caparis, cinamoni ana ℨ iii, mellis quod sufficit, dosis ℨ iiii, cum succo nepito. Antidotum Edmund magistri antedictum, id est, quod datum emagogum,* id est, sanguinem menstrualem ducens, videlicet ad multas mulierum passiones & matricem que non vsu purgantur quia mirabiliter purgat, scilicet mentruales & fetum mortuum in vtero occidit & extrahit & post partum ad sanitatem perducit, petram in vesica frangit & expellit, vrinam mouet, stranguriam sanat, operatur eufrasia† emendit‡ splenis sclirosim & omnia intranea & magnam vtilitatem prestat ad stomachi indignacionem facit; sanat eos qui cibum non continent, flegma fortiter educit & eos curat qui colicam paciuntur neufraticis; prodest homo autem qui vsus fuerit sanitatem optinebit. Cum nil forcius mulieribus inuenitur que illis sunt vtilia. Propter quod cauendum est pacientibus emoroydas aut fluxum matricis aut dissenteriam emoroydas prouocat; vias totius corporis aperit & fetum mortuum & secundinam extrahit & vesicam purgat, stomacum calefacit, vomitum compescit, ventositatem consumit.

*Ad restringuendum coytum*: R$_x$: olei ℨ iiii, camphore ℨ iii, pulverizata camphora; & misceantur et vnge renes & castitatem seruabit. Item, si quis comedit florem salicis vel populi omnem ardorem libidinis in eo refrigerabit bene hoc longo vsu. Item veruena portata vel portata non sinit virgam erigi donec deponatur & si sub seruicali posueris non potest erigi virga vii diebus, quod si probare volueris da gallo mixtam cum furfure & super gallinas non ascendet. [f. 227r] Item herba columbina in testiculo extinguit libidinem. Item inunge corrigiam aliquam cum succo veruene & porta ad carnem & eris effeminatus; & si quam tetigerit erit ineptus ad talia quia cor tangentis emollit. Item lapis sulpicis portata in sinistra manu ereccionem virge tollit. Item testiculi galli cum sanguine suo suppositi lectum coitum iacenti in eo vegitant. Item semen lactuce exsiccat sperma & sedat

*emagogum: MS. emagodum.
†eufrasia: MS. eufraxim.
‡emendit: MS. omendit.

some fleawort, 2 drachms and 1 scruple of purified peonies, 2 drachms of cloves, 3 drachms each of roots of caper and cinnamon, honey as sufficient in portions of 4 drachms, with juice of catmint. The before-mentioned remedy of Master Edmund is the giving of a hemagoge, that is to say, a remedy that causes the flow of menstrual blood; for the many ailments of women and of the womb that are not usually purged, it is a marvelous purge. It purges the menstrual blood, and it kills the dead fetus in the uterus and expels it, and is conducive to health after childbirth, breaks the stone in the bladder, and ejects it, causes urination, heals strangury, makes euphrasy work, cures hardening of the spleen, and all things inside, and is most helpful in the case of disorders of the stomach; it cures those who cannot retain their food, vigorously expels phlegm, and cures those who are suffering from the colic disease of the kidneys; it is useful also to a man who wishes to be as healthy as possible. Nothing has been discovered that is more useful to women. For which reason the patients should beware lest it provokes hemorrhoids or flux of the womb or dysentery. It opens the passages of the whole body, brings out a dead fetus and the secundine and purges the bladder, warms the stomach, checks vomiting, destroys flatulence.

*To restrain sexual intercourse.* Take 4 drachms of oil, 3 drachms of camphor, crushed camphor; let them be mixed and anoint the kidneys, and the preparation will preserve chastity. Again, if anyone eat the best part of the willow or poplar he will effectively cool all the lust in himself by continued usage. Again, vervain carried or drunk will not permit the penis to go stiff until it is laid aside, and vervain placed under the pillow makes an erection impossible for seven days, which prescription, if you wish to test, give to a cock mixed with bran, and the cock will not mount the hen. [f. 227r] Again, the herb columbine extinguishes lust in the testicle. Likewise, anoint the shoelaces with the juice of vervain and wear them against the flesh, and you will be effeminate; and if a man touches anyone he will be inept for such things because it weakens the pleasure of touching. Again, brimstone carried in the left hand will take away an erection. Likewise, the testicles of a cock with its blood placed on the bed cause a man to suppress intercourse. Similarly, the seed in lettuce dries the sperm, quietens

desiderium coitus et pollucionem. Item lapis topazius generat castitatem & reprimit venerem. Item succus iusquiami* testiculos invnge calorem & tumocionem & libidinem extinguit. Item lapis ambri portatus dat castitatem. Item semen salicis sumptum libidinem extinguit. Item eruce, rute & agni casti siccentur & puluerizentur & simul comedentur tollent pollucionem.

*De duricia matricis & eius asperitate.* Fomentum aque decoctionis malue vel altee duriciem tollit. Item axungia† anceris & succus purri miscentur & vngantur collum matricis post menstrua contracta; matricem relaxat. Item lollium, mirra, thus album & coctum simul in vino vel in aqua & fumigetur vel vngatur clausam‡ matricem aperit & ad conceptum disponit. Isaac. Item radix ellebori elixata & fomentata omnem dolorem tollit. Item succi neptis clysterium prouocat. Item emplastrum ex nepita ante & retro prius torificata apositum educit matricem. Item vinum decoctionis origani prouocat menstrua. $R_x$: olei *li.* i, colloquintide ʒ i, succum rute ʒ iii, absinthii, pulegii ana ʒ ii & coquantur & cetera.

*De ictaricia varia*: Patena cum succo marrubii bibita curat. Item succus vrtice rubie cum seruisia bibita. Item rasura emboris bibita curat efficienter. Item crocus dissolutus in aqua & potatus sanat statim. Succus camomille datus potui epatis febribus cum aqua calida mire prodest. [f. 227v] Item succus solatri curat ictariciam. Item aqua pilosella bibita vel vinum decoccionis statim sanat. De lapide: succus arthemisie multus & bibitus curat lapidem & frangit. Item betonica cum mulsa & pipere data potui tollit dolorem & lapidem renum & vesice excludit. Item cortex lauri & eius bacce calculos frangit & expellit.

*iusquiami: MS. iuquiami.
† axungia: MS. auxungia.
‡ clausam: MS. clausa.

lasciviousness and the desire for intercourse. Likewise, the stone topaz produces chastity and represses lechery. Again, anoint the testicles with henbane juice and it extinguishes heat, erection, and lust. Similarly, the stone amber, if carried, promotes chastity. Again, willow seed taken extinguishes lust. Likewise, let colewort, rue, and St.-John's-wort be dried and made into powder, and eaten together they put an end to lasciviousness.

*Concerning hardness of the womb and its roughness.* A poultice of distilled water of common or marshmallows takes away hardness. Likewise, let goose fat and leek juice be mixed and let them be used to oil the neck of the womb after menstrual shrinking; this relaxes the womb. Again, cockle, myrrh, white frankincense cooked at the same time in wine or in water; let them be used to fumigate and oil the shut womb so that it will be opened and made ready for conception. Isaac.* Again hellebore root dug up and treated with warm water takes away all pain; an injection of the juice of catmint provokes it. Likewise, a plaster made from catmint previously dried and applied in front and behind draws out the womb. Similarly, wine in a potion of origanum brings on menstruation. Take 1 pound of oil, 1 ounce of colocynth, 3 drachms of juice of rue, 2 drachms each of wormwood and fleawort, and let them be cooked, etc.

*For various jaundices*: A bowlful of juice of horehound† cures when drunk. Likewise, the juice of red nettle drunk with ale. Again, a scraping of ivory drunk cures effectively. So does saffron dissolved in water and drunk cure instantly. Again, juice of camomile given as a drink with warm water wonderfully benefits fevers of the liver. [f. 227v] So, juice of nightshade cures jaundice. Similarly, water drunk with pilewort or wine in a decoction effects an immediate cure.

Concerning the stone: Juice of artemisia mixed with honey and drunk cures the stone and breaks it. Likewise, betony with honey and pepper given as a drink takes away pain and removes the stone from the kidneys and the bladder; the bark and berries of the laurel break small stones and expel them.

* Possibly Isaac Judaeus (ob. 953) who influenced the early Salernitan writers. Alternatively the reference may be to Gen. 20 ff. Because Abimelech stole Abraham's wife, God made the women of Abimelech's family sterile. When Sarah was restored to Abraham, the curse was lifted, and Sarah conceived Isaac.
† Cf. *Macer Floridus*, ed. Frisk, which recommends juice of "horhowne" thrown up the nose (30a).

*Ad stranguiriam & impedimentum vrine.* Fimus bovis cum melle calefactus & appositus multum valet. Item pili leporis vsti & bibiti statim facit mingere. Item iungat patiens iii diebus super vrticas maiores continuis & exsicca & sic liberatur. Item galbanum appositum super ventrem sub vmbelico statim minget. Item radix raffani in vino albo infusa contusa & trita* per noctem & mane collata statim minget. Item radix pentafiloni *li.* i *sem.*, turmentille ℥ vi, terantur & cum† ptisana cocta & bibita statim curat stranguiriam ex calore. Item vesica capre vsta & bibita. Item sotulares porcinas‡ vstas & bibitas curat. Item advellane assate vtuntur contra distillacionem vrine & amigdale comeste. Item folia agni casti posita in lecto soluit ardorem vrine proprietate sua & non racione.

*De inflacione testiculorum.* Farina fabarum cum succo obuli & oleo communi & apposita statim tollit inflacionem & tumorem. Si virga inflatur cera ℥ ii, cum oleo communi ℨ v, & herbe portulace trite & commixte soluit tumorem. Item farina ordii in multa cocta vel vino albo & emplastra tumorem tollit. Item folia iusquiami *li.* i, folia malue *li. sem..*, cocta in aqua et trite & frixate in melle & vino albo tollit tumorem. Item R$_x$: foliorum maluarum *m.* iii, foliorum absinthii *m.* ii, ebuli *m.* i, coquantur in aquis & illa expressa & herbis tritis & cum melle frixatis cum forma emplastri apponatur secundum magistrum Ricardum Marche.

[f. 228r] **De** *tumore mamille pro multitudine lactis.* Fiat defensiuum ex bolo ℨ i, & olio rosarum ℥ iii, aceti & succo solatri apposito. Item farine fabarum cum albumine ouorum quod sufficit. Item radix caulium, menta, farina fabarum cunna apposita, quia singula lac dissoluunt. Item stercus hominis combustus vlcera cancrosa & quasi insanabilia sanat; & portat pollitricum super se, semper super se, quod certissime sanat cancrum. Item stercus caprum cum melle distemperatum fistulam & cancrum interficit & omnem spuriciam aufert.

*infusa, contusa & trita: MS. infusas, rotulas,& tritas.
† cum: MS. eum.
‡ porcinas: MS. porcinos.

*For a painful discharge of urine and hindrance from urination.* Cow dung warmed with honey and applied helps greatly. Again, the hairs of the hare burnt and drunk instantly cause urination. Likewise, let the patient put on himself for three continuous days, common nettles, get himself dried out, and thus he will be freed. Again, galbanum placed on the stomach below the navel causes instant urination. Likewise, the root of cinquefoil, infused in white wine, pounded and ground to powder, applied at night and early morning, immediately causes urination. Likewise, take 1½ pounds of root of cinquefoil, and 6 ounces of septfoil; let them be rubbed and cooked with barley groats, and drunk at once, and the medicine cures a painful discharge from heat. Similarly, goat's bladder burnt and drunk. Again, piglets burnt and drunk heal. Likewise, roasted filberts and almonds eaten are used for incontinence. Also, the leaves of St.-John's-wort placed in the bed dissolve the heat of the urine by the natural property [of the drug] and not by reason.

*Concerning the swelling of the testicles.* Bean meal with juice of dwarf elder and common oil applied takes away at once the swelling and tumor. If the penis is swollen, 2 ounces of wax with 5 drachms of common oil and the herb purslane ground and mixed does away with the swelling. Also, barley meal cooked in mead or white wine and made into a plaster takes away the tumor. Likewise, 1 pound of leaves of henbane, half a pound of leaves of mallows cooked in water, ground, and stewed in honey and white wine take away the tumor. Also, let 3 handfuls of mallow leaves, 2 handfuls of wormwood leaves, and 1 handful of dwarf elder be cooked in water; and this decoction, squeezed out and roasted with ground herbs and honey, be placed in the form of a plaster, according to Master Richard Marche.

[f. 228r] *Concerning tumor of the breast due to copious milk.* Let this be warded off by 1 drachm of Armenian bole, 3 ounces of oil of roses, applied with vinegar and juice of morel; similarly, bean meal with white of egg as necessary; and root of cabbages, mint, bean meal placed on the genitals, because they alone dissolve the milk. Also, man's excrement when burnt cures cancerous ulcers that seem incurable; and let the patient carry the herb venus' hair above him, always above him, because it most certainly cures cancer. Likewise, the dung of a goat mixed with honey destroys fistula and cancer, and takes away all impurities. Also, let the

Item folia iusquiami cocti & triti cum vitellis coctis ouorum & oleo rosarum & apponentur. Item bardanis cocti sub cineribus cum axungia* & melle appositus sanat putridas mamillas & vlcera. Item fimus murum cum aqua inunctum duriciem vberum & dolorem ac tumorem soluit. Item sanguis leporis cum eius coagulo facit concipere bibitus. Ad pestilenciam $R_x$: mirre, pimpernelle, fumiterre, ana ℥ xii, boli ℥ vi, rute ℥ xv, diptani, tormelle, ana ℥ vi, ligni aloe, sandalis, rubie, pulegii, origani, aristologie rotunde, baccarum lauri ana ℥ x, genciane ℥ vi, puluerizentur. Pro omne egritudine oculorum $R_x$: $4^{xx}$ testudinis in numero & feniculi *m.* xii, coquantur in aqua lagenam *sem.* Contra vomitum $R_x$: seminis acedule, coste, berberis, coralli rubei & albi, ossis de corde cerui, psidii, sandalorum, olei,† tormentillis ana ℥ iii, cumini infusi, anisi vsti, mente, rubee, galange, ligni aloe, gariofoli, amomi interioris, cinamoni, zinziberi albi, ana ʒ i, granarum paradisi, amomi, croci, macis, nardi, carui, zedoarie, cucube, piperis longi & nigri, rosarum, rubearum ana ℥ iiii, subtilissime puluerizentur zucarri albi *li.* i, ciconiorum ℥ xii, aque rosarum ℥ vi, & fiat electuarium ingue in modum diacitonicem, id est, confeccio ciconiorum. Probacio vite. $R_x$: foliorum iusquiami, foliorum rute terantur & fiat emplastrum ad tempora & frontem; si dormit saluus erit si non. [f. 228v] $R_x$: chinarum macedonicorum, salgie, rubie, cerfolii, ipie minoris ana ℥ iii, terantur & bibantur cum soua potu, id est, seruisie ℥ iii, hoc tribus diebus mane, videlicet contra vomitum & fastidium‡ tollit & dat appetitum comedenti & cetera. Probatum est de Lyghtfote Gardener quem vxor sua vocat pater, super quem Gardener probatum erat.

*Ad mulieres tantum*:
Fiat fleobotomia sub cauillis cum subfumigacione radicis yris. Fyrst ther must be made hyr a potage, as it is wreten in retencione menstruorum.

*axungia: MS. auxungia.
† olei: MS. oleum.
‡ fastidium: MS. fastigium.

leaves of henbane cooked and pounded be applied with cooked yolks of eggs and oil of roses. Also, an application of burdocks cooked under ashes with lard and honey cures putrid breasts and ulcers. The dung of mice smeared on with water dissolves hardness of the breasts, and pain, and tumor. Also, the blood of a hare with its curdled milk causes conception when drunk.

For the pestilence: Take 12 drachms each of myrrh, pimpernel, and fumitory, 6 drachms of Armenian bole, 15 drachms of rue, 6 drachms each of dittany, and tourmaline, 10 drachms each of wood aloes, sandalwood, madder, fleawort, origanum, round birthwort, and laurel berries, and 6 drachms of gentian, and let them be made into a powder. For all sickness of the eyes, take an eightieth part of a tortoise exactly, and 12 handfuls of fennel cooked in half a flagon of water. To prevent vomiting: take seed of sorrel, costmary, barberry, red and white coral, the scrapings of the intestine of a deer, 3 drachms each of pomegranates, sandalwood, oil, and tourmaline, infused with cumin, burnt with anise, and 1 ounce each of mint, madder, galingale, wood aloes, cloves, the inner parts of tree nightshade, cinnamon, and white ginger, 4 drachms each of grains of paradise, tree nightshade, saffron, mace, spikenard, caraway, zedoary, cucumber, long and black pepper, and red roses, finely powdered with 1 pound of white sugar, 12 drachms of quinces, 6 drachms of water of roses, and have an electuary made in the manner of diacitonicon syrup, that is, an electuary of quinces.

*Testing for life.* Have the leaves of henbane and the leaves of rue ground, made into a plaster, and applied to the temples and forehead: if he sleeps he will be saved, otherwise not. [f. 228v] Take 3 drachms each of Macedonian artichokes, rock salt, madder, chervil, and chickweed, let them be ground and drunk with a mild drink, that is, 3 drachms of ale, every morning for three days, and the decoction is effective against vomiting as it takes away nausea, gives an appetite for eating, etc. This has been tested on Lightfoot the gardener,* whose wife calls him "father," upon which gardener it [the prescription] was tested.

*For women only*: Let a phlebotomy be made under the ankles with a fumigation of the root of iris.

First a soup must be made for her, as is written in the chapter on the retention of menses.

---

* Alternatively, Gardener may be a surname and "lightfoot" either an epithet or adjective meaning light-footed, fleet, qualifying Gardener.

2$^e$: After þat sche muste haue hyr drynke, as it is writen in suffocacione menstruorum.

3$^e$: Sche must haue a pelowe that she must sitte on in bath, writen in suffocacione menstruorum.

4$^e$: Sche muste haue hyr bathe, as it is writen in suffocacione menstruorum.

5: She muste haue an vnguente for hyr lymmes, as it is writen in suffocacione menstruorum.

6: She muste haue suppositories, as it is writen in mola matricis.

7: She muste haue pissaries, as it is writen in mola.

8: She muste haue emplastris for hyr wombe, as it is writen in childing in þe byrthe.

9: She muste haue anoyntyng to bryng forth.

10: She muste haue trociscis of mirr with hyr decoccions of duretyke.

For brakyng: take rosemarie, rede myntes, lorer leves ana ℈ iii & *sem.* clowes ℥ *sem.* Sethe alle these in rede wyne þre quartes of zucre roset ℥ iii, & clense it. A Stuphe: *Take of mugwort, wormewode & nept, origanum, paritorie, puliol,† mounteyn, rue, off yche aliche moche; boyle hem well all togeder [f. 229r] in water and make a stuphe. A drynk: Take also wyne þat comyn and parsely rotes & mugwort, of rotes of pestnepe of þe felde & rotes of gladyn boyled in with hony a sawser full clarified. Anoþer drynk: Take mugwort, diptayne, savyne, englyssh mader, pyonye, of yche aliche moche & stampe hem & boile hem in Osy wyne or bastard & put þerto clarified hony & drynk it ofte with pouder of jete.

A plastre: Take leves of marygulde, chykmete, paritorie & stampe hem with þe sedes of gromyll & of columbyne, with xii pepercornes, make a plastre and drynke of herbes.‡

Divers tymes it happith of diuers women a mischeuous greuaunce in trauaillinge of chyld for defaute of good mydwifes, and that greuaunce kepen priue & it nedith for to be holpen. To summe women happith this greuaunce: þat þe peritoneon brekith, þat þer is but oon issue for bothe voydaunces. And of these women ofte tymes comith out þe marice for þe weye is made so large in her trauaylyng & so þe marice waxith harde &

*MS. margin: secundum Edmond prester.
† puliol: MS. piliol.
‡ herbes: MS. herbes a plastre.

Second: After that she must have her potion, as is written in the chapter on the repression of menses.

Third: She must have a pillow that she can sit on in the bath, as is written in the chapter on the repression of menses.

Fourth: She must have her bath, as is written in the chapter on the repression of menses.

5: She must have an unguent for her limbs, as is described in the suppression of menstruation.

6: She must have suppositories, as is described in the mola of the womb.

7: She must have pessaries, as is written in [the chapter on] mola.

8: She must have plasters for her womb, as is written in [the chapter on] childbirth.

9: She must be anointed with oils in order to give birth.

10: She must have myrrh pills with her potions of diuretic.

For vomiting: Take 3   drachms each of rosemary, red mint, laurel leaves, and half an ounce of cloves. Boil all these in 3 quarts of red wine and 3 ounces of rose sugar, and strain.

A bath: Take an equal amount of mugwort, wormwood, catmint, origanum, pellitory, wild thyme, and rue; boil them all well together [f. 229r] in water and make a bath.

A drink: Take also wine in which cumin, parsley roots, mugwort, roots of field parsnip, and roots of iris are boiled in with a saucer of clear honey.

Another drink: Take mugwort, dittany, savin, English madder, peony, of each an equal amount, crush them, boil them in Ozey or Bastard wine,* and add to the mixture clarified honey, and drink it often with jet powder.

A plaster: Take marigold leaves, chickweed, and pellitory, grind them with the seeds of gromwell, columbine, and 12 peppercorns, make a plaster and drink of herbs.

On numerous occasions, different women experience great distress in giving birth through lack of a good midwife, and that distress is kept secret, and it requires assistance. Some women have this problem: the peritoneum breaks, so that there is only one outlet for both evacuations. And in these women sometimes the womb comes out because the aperture has been made so large during labor, and so the womb grows hard and will not

---

* Both well-known sweetened wines.

wyll not be sette ayen in her owne place but yf it be holpen be medecyn. And þe helthe muste be in þis maner. Take good whyȝt wyne & make it hoote & putt butter in þat wyne þat be fresshe & not salt & with wyne softely moiste þe marice ofte tymes till it wexe souple & softe & þanne esilich putt it into þe membre ther it shulde be. And after that, sewe þe breche of þe peritoneon in thre places or foure with a double silken threde; thanne putt a lynnen cloute into þe membre after þe quantite of þe membre, scilicet vulue. And after þat lyne it aboue with [f. 229v] hote tarre & þat shall make þe marice withdrawe & so sitt faste for þe stynkyng of þe tarre & þan shall þe breche be heled & yclosed with pouder of confery & of petyt consowe & of canell. And ley þe pacient in hir bedde vpright so þat her fete lye heyher þan her hede & lete hyr lyen so ix dayes and so without remevyng fro thens, do her nedys. And make her ete liquide metes mesurabelich in þat seson & drynk also. And after ix dayes ben passed, make hyr arise & mesurabelich let her kepe herself fro trauaylle or besynesse, & she mote kepe her from bathes & from all metes þat ben evyll to defyen & fro hevy metes & fro suche metis as wyl engendre þe cough. Also it is for to wete þat þer muste be putt into þe arshole a tywel made of a lynnen cloute to stoppe þat þe egestion goo not out but whan tyme of voydaunce ben in þe ix dayes forsaid.

There be also other women in þe whiche ofte tymes her marice wyl come doun & summe tyme arise for summe cause, & hit ben such women þat mowe not suffre a mannes yerde for þe gretnesse þerof, & summe tyme þey be constreyned to suffre wyl they nyl they. To suche women we put þe medecyn forsaid of þe lynnen clout with þe tarre. And yf we haue no tarre, we take a lynnen clout & moysten it with oleo hote of puliole or muscelyn & we putt it into þe membre, scilicet vulua, & we bynde it there till þe marice be setled. And þe women be forbede metes þat shuld make hem to cogh, & drynk also. Also it is to wite þat þe comyng out of þe marice in an olde woman is incurable; and also in a yong woman yf it come out with moche blode & so haue be longe tyme duryng. But þat [f. 230r] that hath not long tyme dured may be holpen þus. At þe begynnyng we muste moiste þe marice with þe water þat malowes & þe holyhok was soden in. And after þat we anoynt þe membra, scilicet vulua, with aragon

be fixed again in its own place unless assisted by medicine. And the cure is this: Take good white wine, make it hot, add butter that is fresh and not salt, and with the wine gently moisten the womb many times until it grows supple and soft, and then gently put the womb into the place where it should be. And after that, sew up the breach of the peritoneum in three or four places with a double silken thread. Then put a linen cloth into the part, that is to say, the vulva, according to its size. And afterward cover it with [f. 229v] hot tar, and that will make the womb withdraw and thus remain firm because of the evil smell of the tar, and then the breach will be healed and closed with powder of comfrey, little daisy, and cinnamon. And place the patient upright in her bed, so that her feet are higher than her head, and let her remain for nine days and, thus keeping her in bed, attend to her needs. And make her eat liquid foods moderately at that time and drink also. And after nine days have passed, make her get up and let her within moderation keep herself from work or business, and she must refrain from baths, and all foods that are difficult to digest, and from heavy foods, and from such food as will promote coughing. And it is necessary to know that a linen towel must be put into the anus to prevent evacuation except at time of excretion in the nine days already mentioned.

There are also other women whose womb often will come down and then sometimes go up for some reason, and such women cannot endure a man's penis because of the size of it, and sometimes they are forced to endure it whether they would or not. We give the previously mentioned medicine of the linen rag with tar to such women.* And if we have no tar, we take a linen rag and moisten it with hot oil of wild thyme or musk, and we put it into the part, that is to say, the vulva, and we fasten it there until the womb has settled. And the women should be forbidden foods that make them cough, and also drink. Also, it is necessary to know that in an old woman the coming out of the womb is incurable; and also in a young woman, if it comes out with much blood and is of long duration. But a condition [f. 230r] that has not lasted long may be helped thus. At the beginning we must moisten the womb with water that mallows and hollyhock have been boiled in. After that, we anoint the part, that is, the vulva, with aragon

* A kind of proto-diaphragm.

& þe share also; and also with marciaton & oleo of puliole & so we put in ayen þe marice. And þan we make the woman sitte on a sege wel closed with clothes and þan vnder þe sege with hote coles. And we putt on þe coles stynkyng thynges as cloutes of wolle & heer and stynkyng herbes as homelok & suche oþer and so shall þe marice abyde in her place. And whan þe marice is þus inne, we make a plastre vpon þe sharis of mastyk & frankencence & bole armoniak & sankdragon & picche medled togedre & þat kepith it euermore stille. Yff so be a woman desire to conceyue of a man that she wold conceyve of, it muste first be wyst yf she be able to haue her desire, þat is for to wyten yf ony defaute be of one of hem or of bothe. Thus it may be wist: take twey litell pottes as hit were mustard pottes & in yche of þe pottes putte whete branne; & put of þe mannes vryne in þat oon potte and of þe womannes vryne in þat oþer potte & so late þe pottes stonde ix dayes or more. And yf cas be þat þe man be not able, þou shalt fynde after tho ix daies wormes in þe vryne and foule stynkyng. And yf þe defaute be in þe woman, þou shalt fynde þe same proof. And yf wormes appere not in neyther vryne, thorough medecynes they mow be amendid & haue her desyre with þe grace of God as þus: take þe stones of a bore & drye hem in a potte closed with a couercle wel litell or prassed aboute þe joyntures þat noon eyrs [f. 230v] come out in an ovene; whanne þei be dried make poudre þerof & let þe woman drynk þerof, after þat she is purged.

*De floribus.* And þan late her come & she shall conceyve with þe grace of god. But she muste drynk þat pouder with good wyn; and yf she desire to conceyue a male child, they muste take þe marice of an hare & þe cunt, and dryen it in þe forsaid manere & poudren it & drink þe pouder þerof with wyne. And yf þe woman desire a femel childe, lete her drye þe stones of an hare & in þe ende of her floures, make pouder þerof and drynk þerof to bedde wardes & þan go pley with her make. Another medecyn for a woman þat may not conceyve: take þe stones & þe lyuer of a pigge þat is deliuered of a sowe allone and make poudre þerof, & gyve þe woman to drynke with wyne whan she gothe to bedde to her make, & she shall conveyve, witnesse Trotula.

A medecyn for þe stone proued trewe:

Take þe sedes of gromell, careway, parcely, saxifrage, fenell, lufache, smalache, stanmarche, and cherystone kernell, rotes of filipendula, of iche of these aliche moche of weight. And make pouder of hit & drynke

and we anoint the genitals also; and also with ointment and oil
of thyme, and thus we put the womb in again. And then we
make the woman sit on a seat well covered with cloths with hot
coals under it. And we put evil-smelling things such as wool
rags, hair, and foul-smelling herbs such as hemlock, and similar
things on the coals, and as a result the womb will stay in its
place. And when the womb is thus in its place, we make a plaster
upon the genitals of mastic, frankincense, Armenian bole, sandragon and pitch mixed together, and that fixes it for good. If a
woman desires to conceive, it must first be ascertained whether
she is able to have her wish, to know if there is any fault in either
one of them or both. It may be ascertained thus: Take 2 little
pots like mustard pots, and in each of the pots put wheat bran;
and put the man's urine in one pot and the woman's in the other
pot, and so let the pots stand nine or more days. And if the fault
is in the man, after those nine days you will find worms in the
urine and a terrible smell. And if the fault is in the woman, you
will find the same proof. And if worms appear in neither pot of
urine, the condition of the man and the woman can be remedied,
and they may have their wish with the grace of God through
medicines thus: Take the testicles of a boar and dry them in a pot
closed by a lid very small or pressed about the joints so that no
fumes [f. 230v] come out in an oven; when the testicles are
dried, make a powder of them and let the woman drink it, after
which she will have her purgation.

*Concerning menstruation.* And then let her come and she will
conceive with God's grace. But she must drink that powder with
good wine; and if she wishes to conceive a male child, the man
and woman must take the womb of a hare and its pudendum,
dry it in the way previously mentioned, powder it, and drink the
powder of it with wine. And if the woman desires a female child,
let her dry the testicles of a hare, and at the end of her menstrual
period make a powder of it, drink it at bedtime, and then go to
play with her mate. Another medicine for a woman unable to
conceive: Take the testicles and liver of a pig that has given birth
to a single sow, make powder of it, and give the woman it to
drink in wine when she goes to her husband in bed, and she will
conceive, as Trotula testifies.

A tested medicine for the stone: Take the seeds of gromwell,
caraway, parsley, saxifrage, fennel, lovage, smallage, horse-
parsley, cherrystone kernel, roots of dropwort, an equal
amount of each. And make a powder and have the patient drink

a sponefull at ones of þe pouder in whyt wyne or ale ywarmed fyrst & last till she be all hole. And yf it be vsed in potage, it worchith þe better. And yf ye haue þe colyk,* putte to þe poudre of bayes of þe lorere half as moche in weight as of oone of þe forsayd sedes.

Anoþer medecyne for þe stoone:

Take rotes of parcely, rotes of fenell, rotes of smalache, rotes of radych, rotes of gromyll, rotes [f. 231r] of saxifrage, rotes of alisaunder, rotes of filipendula—of eche an handfull; fenell seed, parcely seed, smallache seed, loveache, carewey seed, gromel sede, saxifrage sede, kyrnells of cherystones, alisaundre seed—of iche an ounce; cinamome† half an ounce; bray all these a litell & boyle hem in þre potell of water to a potell with esy fyre, þe vessell ycouered, & whan it is colde, strayne out þe licour & medle þerwith iiij ounces of sugre & boyle hem a while togeders. And þen þere is a drynke of þe whyche vse by þe morewe first; at nyght last a good draught mylke warme. $R_x$: benedicte ʒ i, interiorum colloquintidis ʒ sem., hermodactilis Ð ii, pulveris dominici, diamargariton ana Ð sem., fiant pelli cum aqua argillis‡ vel spigernillis. And this medecyne aforne writen is good to dissoluen þe colyk.

A good medecyn for þe palsy: Fyrst take primerolles, wylde sauge, straweberiwise, folefote leves—of eche a good handfull and hak hem right small & þan boyle hem, yif it be for a man, in a potell of barowes grece. And yf it be for a woman in a potell of sowe grece, & boyle all togeder with a gret sokyng fyre fyve or foure oures at þe leste. And þan late it stonde all nyght in þe potte þat it is boyled yn. And in þe morewetide, hete it & drawe it thorough a streynour, and kepe it in a close vessel. And it will kepe itself vi or vii yere good ynogh. And ley þe syke ayen þe fyre, nout to hote; and anoynt þe sike twyes on þe day there he is disesed vpon the joyntes.

A medecyn for þe palsye:

[f. 231v] Take peletre of Spayne, erbe benet, anneys, parcely, galyngale, clowes, notemuge, sauge, rewe, stanmarche, maces, Frenche sene, þe sede of a best þat is called castory, and longe peper ana yliche moche—an ounce yf þou wilt or els more or lasse—& make hem all togedre in a poudre. And sarce hem clene and ete of þat pouder half a sponefull in þi

*MS.: And yf ye have þe have þe colyk.

† cinamome: MS. omamome.

‡ argillis: MS. ardillis.

a spoonful of the powder at one go in white wine or warmed ale first thing in the morning and last thing at night until she is cured. And if it is used in soup, it works all the better. And if you have the colic, add to the powder the fruit of the laurel tree half as much in weight as one of the previously mentioned seeds.

Another medicine for the stone: Take roots of parsley, fennel, smallage, radish, gromwell, [f. 231r] saxifrage, horse-parsley, dropwort, a handful of each; 1 ounce each of seed of fennel, parsley, smallage, lovage, caraway, gromwell, saxifrage, cherrystone kernels, horse-parsley seed, and half an ounce of cinnamon; crush all these a little and boil them in 1½ gallons of water to half a gallon on a gentle fire, the pot covered, and when it is cold strain it, mix it with 4 ounces of sugar, and boil for a time together. This potion you should use first thing in the morning; last thing at night have a good draft of warm milk. Take 1 drachm of benedicta, half a drachm of the inner parts of the colocynth, 2 scruples of colchicum, half a scruple each of *pulveris dominici*, perforated and nonperforated pearls, and let pills be made with water, argil, or spigurnel,* and the aforesaid medicine is good to cure the colic.

A good medicine for the palsy: First take primroses, wild sage, strawberry plants, coltsfoot leaves—of each a good handful, chop them very small, and then boil them, if the medicine is for a man, in half a gallon of boar's grease. And if the medicine is for a woman, in half a gallon of sow's grease, and boil them all together on a great slow fire at least four or five hours. And then let it stand all night in the pot in which it is boiled. And the next day, heat it, strain it, and keep it in a closed container. And it will keep well enough six or seven years. And place the sick person near a moderate fire; and anoint him twice a day on the affected joints.

A medicine for the palsy: [f. 231v] Take pellitory of Spain hemlock, anise, parsley, galingale, cloves, nutmeg, sage, rue, horse-parsley, mace, French senna, dried glands of beaver, that is, castory, and long pepper in an equal amount—an ounce, if you wish, or more or less—and make them all into a powder. And strain them clean, and eat half a spoonful of that powder in your

* See *O.E.D.* s.v. *spigurnel* (1).

potage afore mete. And yche day duryng þi lyf wassche thy necke & þi handes and all thy ioyntes of þyne armes with aqua vite, and yche thyrde day drynk a sponefull of aqua vite after thy mete.

For to make aqua vite aforesaid:

First take ii galons of þe strengest wyne þat þou may gete & put it in a clene vessell & put þerto origanum & lauendre & tyme, rosemary & sawge, wyldesauge, puliole mountayne, puliole riall, primerolles, couselippes, carlokkis—of eche even porcion; of poudre of castory aforesaid di *li*, & a potel of gret mustard. And put all these & þe wyne into a vessell & stylle it vp in two stillatories & vse it as it is before said. A medecyn for þe palsie þat makith a man to tremble: Take rede fenell and parcely, saveyn, lorer leves—of eche an handfull—and an half handfull of whyȝt malues and another of radyssh, and a handfull of avence and ii handfull of primerolles & an *m*. of lauendre & anoþer of isop & anoþer of borage & anoþer of croppes of reed netles, & ij *m*. of betayn and ij handful of hertis tunge and ij of solsequium & an *m*. of violet & another of waterkersen. And also moche of sauge as halfen dele thyne other herbes amounten be weight. And þanne [f. 232r] lete wasshe hem riȝt clene and stampe hem and than do hem into a newe erthen potte and do þerto a galon of fyne rede wyne and þre potellis of fyne sprynging water and do þerto a potell of fyne lyf hony that is boyled and wel eskomed; and þanne sethe alle þese well togeders till þat þei come to a galon and þan take it downe of the fyre and streyne it þorogh a streynour and do hit in a feyre clene vessell and kover it right well and lete þe seke vse of þat drynk first and laste—at even hote and atte morewen cold—tyll he be hoole of þat maladie.

soup before food. And every day of your life wash your neck, hands, and all the joints in your arms with *aqua vitae*, and every third day drink a spoonful of *aqua vitae* after your food.

To make the previously mentioned *aqua vitae*: First take 2 gallons of the strongest wine that you can procure, put it in a clean pan, and add to it origanum, lavender, thyme, rosemary, sage, wild sage, mountain thyme, thyme, primroses, cowslips, charlocks—an equal amount of each; add half a pound of castory powder previously mentioned, and half a gallon of large-leaved mustard. Put all these and the wine in a pot, distill it in 2 stills, and use it as previously prescribed.

A medicine for the palsy, a disease which makes a man shake: Take red fennel, parsley, savin, laurel leaves—a handful of each—half a handful of white mallows and another of radishes, a handful of harefoot, 2 handfuls of primroses, a handful each of lavender, hyssop, borage, and shoots of red nettles, 2 handfuls each of betony, hart's-tongue, heliotrope, a handful of violets and another of watercress, and also as much sage as half the weight of the rest of the herbs put together. And then [f. 232r] have them well washed, pound them, place them in a new earthen pot, and add a gallon of fine red wine, 1½ gallons of fine spring water, and then half a gallon of fine liquid honey, boiled and well skimmed; and then boil all these well together until they come to a gallon, and then take the pan off the fire, strain the liquid through a strainer, place it in a fine clean container, cover it well, and let the patient use that drink first thing in the morning and last thing at night—hot in the evening and cold in the morning—until he be cured of that sickness.

# BIBLIOGRAPHY

This bibliography lists the printed works consulted—medical, theological, historical, literary, and others. It is not intended as a comprehensive bibliography of books, articles, and other texts pertaining to the study of medieval gynecology.

*Aetios of Amida*. Trans. James V. Ricci. Phildelphia: Blackiston, 1950.

Albertus Magnus. *Opera Omnia*. Ed. A. Borgnet. 38 vols. Paris, 1890–99.

————. *Book of Minerals*. Trans. Dorothy Wykoff. Oxford: Clarendon Press, 1967.

Albucasis. *Gynaecia*. See Wolff.

Amundsen, Darrel W. "Medieval Canon Law on Medical and Surgical Practice by the Clergy." *Bulletin of the History of Medicine*, 52 (1978), 22–44.

Arderne, John. *Treatises of Fistula in Ano*. Ed. D'Arcy Power, Early English Text Soc., Original Series, 139. 1910; rpt. London: Oxford Univ. Press, 1969.

Aristotle. *Generation of Animals*. Trans. A. L. Peck. Loeb ed. London: Heinemann, 1943.

*Aristotle's Masterpiece or the Secrets of Generation*. London: F. L. for J. How, 1690.

Arnaldus de Villanova. *Breviarium Practice*. Lyons, 1509. See also Sigerist.

St. Augustine. "De Genesi ad Litteram." *Patrologia Latina*. Vol. 34. Ed. J.-P. Migne. Paris, 1887.

Aveling, J. H. *English Midwives; Their History and Prospects* [1872]. Introd. John L. Thornton. London: Hugh K. Elliott, 1967.

————. "An Account of the Earliest English Work on Midwifery and the Diseases of Women." *Obstetrical Journal of Great Britain and Ireland*, 14 (1874), 73–83.

Baker, A. T. "La Vie de Saint Edmond." *Romania*, 55 (1929), 332–81.

Ballantyne, J. W. "The 'Byrth of Mankynde'." *The Journal of Obstetrics and Gynaecology of the British Empire*, 10 (1906), 297–325.

Barrough, Philip. *The Method of Physick*. London, 1653.

Bartholomaeus Anglicus. *De Proprietatibus rerum*. 1601; rpt. Frankfurt: Minerva, 1964.

Bayon, H. P. "Trotula and the Ladies of Salerno." *Proceedings of the Royal Society of Medicine*, 33 (1939–40), 471–75.

Bernardino, St. *Opera Omnia*. 9 vols. Florence: Guarrachi, 1950–65.

*Bevis of Hampton*. Ed. E. Kölbing, Early English Text Soc., Extra Series, 46, 48, 65. London: Trübner, 1885–94.

176

Bonner, Campbell. *Studies in Magical Amulets, Chiefly Graeco-Egyptian.* Ann Arbor: Univ. of Michigan Press, 1950.

Bracton, Henry de. *De Legibus et Consuetudinibus Angliae.* Ed. George E. Woodbine. 1922; rpt. Cambridge, Mass.: Harvard Univ. Press, 1968.

Budge, E. A. *Amulets and Superstitions.* London: Oxford Univ. Press, 1930.

Bühler, Curt F. "Prayers and Charms in Certain Middle English Scrolls." *Speculum,* 39 (1964), 270–78.

Bullough, Vern L. "Medieval Medical and Scientific Views of Women." *Viator,* 4 (1973), 485–501.

Celsus, Aurelius Cornelius. *Of Medicine, in Eight Books.* Trans. James Grieve. London: D. Wilson and T. Durham, 1756.

———. *De Medicina.* Trans. W. G. Spencer. 3 vols. London: Heinemann, 1935–38.

*Chartularum universitatis Parisiensis.* 4 vols. Ed. P. Heinrich Denifle. Paris: Delalain, 1889–97.

Chesnel, Adolphe de. *Dictionnaire des Superstitions, erreurs, préjugés, et traditions populaires.* Petit-Montrouge: J. P. Migne, 1856.

Cholmeley, H. P. *John of Gaddesden and the "Rosa Medicinae."* Oxford: Clarendon, 1912.

Clay, Rotha Mary. *The Mediaeval Hospitals of England.* 1909; rpt. London: Cass, 1966.

Constantinus Africanus, *De Coitu.* Trans. Paul Delany. *Chaucer Review,* 4 (1970), 55–65.

Cronin, H. S. "The Twelve Conclusions of the Lollards." *English Historical Review,* 22 (1907), 295–304.

Culpepper, Nicholas. *Culpepper's Compleat and Experienc'd Midwife in Two Parts.* Made English by W-S- M.D. 3rd. ed. London: n.p., 1718.

*Customary of Benedictine Monasteries of St. Augustine, Canterbury, and St. Peter, Westminster.* 2 vols. Ed. E. Maunde Thompson. London: Henry Bradshaw Society, nos. 23, 27, 1902, 1904.

Delcourt, Joseph, ed. *Medicina de Quadrupedibus.* Heidelberg: Winter, 1914.

Denifle, P. Heinrich. *Die Entstehung der Universitäten des Mittelalters bis 1400.* Berlin: Weidmann, 1885.

De Renzi, S. *Collectio Salernitana.* 5 vols. Naples: Filiatre-Sebezio, 1852–59.

Dioscorides. *Pedanii Dioscuridis Anazarbei de Materia Medica Libri Quinque.* Ed. Max Wellmann. 3 vols. Berlin: Weidmann, 1907–14.

Donceel, Joseph F. "Immediate Animation and Delayed Hominization." *Theol. Stud.,* 31 (1970), 78–85.

Drabkin, Miriam F., and Israel E. Drabkin, eds. *Caelius Aurelianus: Gynaecia.* Baltimore: Johns Hopkins, 1941.

Dubois, Pierre. *De Recuperatione Terre Sancte, Traité de politique générale par Pierre Dubois.* Ed. Ch.-V. Langlois. Paris: Picard, 1891.

Edmund, St. See Baker; Lawrence; Ward.

Engbring, G. M. "Saint Hildegard, Twelfth-Century Physician." *Bulletin of the History of Medicine*, 8 (1940), 770–84.

*English Mediaeval Lapidaries*. Ed. J. Evans and M. S. Sergeantson. Early English Text Soc., Original Series, 190. 1933; rpt. London: Oxford Univ. Press, 1960.

*The English Register of Godstow Nunnery, near Oxford*. Ed. A. Clark. Early English Text Soc., Original Series, 129, 130, 142. London: Kegan Paul, 1905–11.

Findley, Palmer. "The Midwives' Books." *Medical Life*, 42 (1935), 167–86.

Flemming, Percy. "The Medical Aspects of the Mediaeval Monastery in England." *Proceedings of the Royal Society of Medicine*, 22 (1928–29), 771–82.

*Fleta*. Ed. H. G. Richardson and G. O. Sayles. 4 vols. London: Seldon Soc., 1955–72.

Forbes, T. R. *The Midwife and the Witch*. New Haven and London: Yale Univ. Press, 1966.

Frère, W. H., ed. *Visitation Articles and Injunctions*. 3 vols. Alcuin Club, 14–16. London: Longmans, 1910.

Galen, Claudius. *Claudii Galeni Opera Omnia*. 20 vols. Ed. C. G. Kühn. Leipzig: n.p., 1821–33.

——. *On the Natural Faculties*. Trans. Arthur John Brock. Loeb ed. London: Heinemann, 1963.

——. *De Usu Partium*. Ed. G. Helmreich. 2 vols. 1907–9; rpt. Amsterdam: Hakkert, 1968.

*Gammer Gurton's Needle*. Ed. J. S. Farmer. London: Gibbins, 1906.

Garbáty, T. J. "Chaucer's Weaving Wife." *Journal of American Folklore*, 81 (1968), 342–46.

Gilbertus Anglicus. *Compendium Medicine*. Lyons: Iacobus Saccon for V. de Portonariis, 1510.

Godefroy, F. *Dictionnaire de l'ancienne Langue Française*. 10 vols. Paris: Vieweg, 1881–1902.

Gourevitch, Danielle. "Pudeur et Practique Médicale dans l'antiquité classique." *Presse Médicale*, 76 (1968), 544–46.

Gower, John. *The Complete Works of John Gower*. Ed. G. C. Macaulay. 4 vols. Oxford: Clarendon Press, 1899–1902.

Gray, Douglas. "Notes on Some Middle English Charms." In *Chaucer and Middle English Studies in Honour of Rossell Hope Robbins*. Ed. Beryl Rowland. London: Allen & Unwin, 1974.

Grindal, Edmund. *The Remains of Edmund Grindal*. Ed. W. Nicholson. Cambridge: Cambridge Univ. Press, 1843.

Guy de Chauliac. *The Cyrurgie of Guy de Chauliac*. Ed. Margaret Ogden. Early English Text Soc., 265. London: Oxford Univ. Press, 1971.

Halliwell, J. O. *A Dictionary of Archaic and Provincial Words*. 2 vols. London: Smith, 1847.

Hamilton, George L. "Trotula." *Modern Philology*, 4 (1906), 377–80.

Handerson, Henry E. *Gilbertus Anglicus. Medicine of the Thirteenth Century*. Cleveland, Ohio: CMLA, 1918.

Hargreaves, Henry. "De spermate hominis." *Mediaeval Studies*, 39 (1977), 506–10.

Harris, Walter. *A Treatise of the Acute Diseases of Infants . . . written originally in Latin by the late learned Walter Harris M.D.* Trans. John Martin. London: Thomas Astley, 1742.

Heinrich, F., ed. *Ein mittelenglisches Medizinbuch*. Halle, 1896.

Henslow, G. *Medical Works of the Fourteenth Century*. London: Chapman & Hall, 1899.

Hildegard, St. "Liber Subtilitatum." *Patrologia Latina*. Vol. 197. Ed. J. P. Migne. Paris, 1882.

———. "Vita Sanctae Hildegardis." Ibid.

———. *Causae et curae*. Ed. Paul Kaiser. Leipzig: Teubner, 1903.

Hippocrates. *Oeuvres Complètes d'Hippocrate*. Trans. E. Littré. 10 vols. Paris: Ballière, 1839–61.

Höfler, M. *Volksmedizin und Aberglaube*. Munich: Otto Galler, 1893.

Horton-Smith Hartley, P., and H. R. Aldridge. *Johannes de Mirfeld of St. Bartholomew's Smithfield. His Life and Works*. Cambridge: Cambridge Univ. Press, 1936.

Hübner, Aemilius. *Inscriptiones Hispaniae Latinae*. Berlin: Reimer, 1869.

Hughes, Muriel Joy. *Women Healers in Medieval Life and Literature*. 1943; rpt. New York: Books for Libraries, 1968.

Hurd-Mead, Kate Campbell. *A History of Women in Medicine*. Haddam, Conn.: Haddam Press, 1938.

Hyginus. *Hygini Fabulae*. Ed. M. Schmidt. Jena: H. Dufft, 1872.

Ilberg, Johannes. *Die Überlieferung der Gynäkologie des Soranos von Ephesos*. Leipzig: Teubner, 1911.

Ingerslev, E. "Rösslin's Rosegarten: Its Relation to the Past (the Muscio Manuscripts and Soranos), Particularly with Regard to Podalic Version." *Journal of Obstetrics and Gynaecology of the British Empire*, 15 (1909), 1–25; 73–92.

*Irish Texts, Fasciculus V*, ed. J. Fraser, P. Grosjean, and J. G. O'Keefe. London: Sheed and Ward, 1934.

James, Montague Rhodes. *The Ancient Libraries of Canterbury and Dover. The Catalogues of the Libraries of Christchurch Priory and St. Augustine's Abbey at Canterbury and St. Martin's Priory at Dover*. Cambridge: Cambridge Univ. Press, 1903.

Jonas, Richard. *The Byrth of Mankynde*. London: T. R., 1540.

Jones, Ida B. "Popular Medical Knowledge in Fourteenth-Century English Literature." *Bulletin of the Institute of the History of Medicine*, 5 (1937), 405–51; 538–88.

Josephus. *The Works of Flavius Josephus*. Trans. W. Whiston. 2 vols. London: Bohn, 1845.

Kane, Elisha Kent, ed. *The Book of Good Love by Juan Ruiz*. Introd. John Esten Keller. Chapel Hill, N.C.: Univ. of North Carolina Press, 1968.

Kibre, Pearl. "The Faculty of Medicine at Paris, Charlatanism, and Unlicensed Medical Practices in the Later Middle Ages." *Bulletin of the History of Medicine*, 27 (1953), 1–20.

Kriegk, G. L. *Deutsches Bürgerthum im Mittelalter.* 2 vols. 1871; rpt. Frankfurt: Sauer & Auvermann K. G., 1969.

Kristeller, Paul Oskar. "The School of Salerno." *Bulletin of the History of Medicine*, 17 (1945), 138–94.

Kuppe, G. "Zwillingskollision mit Kinn-zu-Kinn-Verhakung." *Zentralblatt fuer Gynaekologie*, 95 (1973), 583–86.

Lawn, Brian. *The Salernitan Question.* Oxford: Clarendon Press, 1963.

Lawrence, C. H. *St. Edmund of Abingdon.* Oxford: Clarendon Press, 1960.

Le Clerc, Daniel. *Histoire de la Médicine.* La Haye: Vanderkloot, 1729.

Lipinska, Mélanie. *Histoire des Femmes Médicins depuis l'Antiquité jusqu'à nos Jours.* Paris: Jacques, 1900.

*Macer Floridus de Viribus Herbarum, A Middle English Translation of.* Ed. Gösta Frisk. 1949; rpt. Nendeln/Liechtenstein: Kraus, 1973.

MacKinney, Loren C. "Medieval Medical Dictionaries and Glossaries." *Medieval and Historiographical Essays in Honor of James Westfall Thompson.* Ed. James Cate and E. Anderson. Chicago: Univ. of Chicago Press, 1938.

———. "Childbirth in the Middle Ages as Seen in Manuscripts." *Ciba Symposium*, 8 (1960), 230–36.

———. *Medical Illustrations in Medieval Manuscripts.* Berkeley and Los Angeles: Univ. of California Press, 1965.

Martial. *Epigrams.* Trans. Walter C. Ker. Loeb ed. 2 vols. London: Heinemann, 1961.

Mason-Hohl, Elizabeth. See Trotula.

Matthews, William. "The Wife of Bath and All her Sect." *Viator*, 5 (1974), 413–43.

Maubray, John. *The Female Physician.* London: John Holland, 1724.

Meyer, C. F. "A Middle English Leech Book and its XIV Century Poem on Bloodletting." *Bulletin of the History of Medicine*, 7 (1939), 388–90.

Meyer, Paul. "Recettes Médicales en Provençal." *Romania*, 32 (1903), 268–99.

*Middle English Dictionary.* Ed. Hans Kurath and Sherman M. Kuhn. Ann Arbor, Mich.: Univ. of Michigan Press, 1954.

Mirfeld, John. See Horton-Smith.

Mondeville, Henri de. *Chirurgie de Maître Henri de Mondeville.* Paris: Ballière, 1893.

Myrc, John. *Instructions for Parish Priests by John Myrc.* Ed. Edward Peacock; trans. F. J. Furnivall. Early English Text Soc., Original Series, 31. 1902; rpt. New York: Greenwood, 1969.

*The Myroure of oure Ladye.* Ed. John Henry Blunt. Early English Text Soc., Extra Series, 19. London: Trübner, 1873.

Noonan, J. T., Jr. *Contraception: A History of its Treatment by the Catholic Theologians and Canonists.* Cambridge, Mass.: Harvard Univ. Press, 1966.

————. "Abortion and the Catholic Church: A Summary History." *Natural Law Forum*, 12 (1967), 88–131.

————, ed. *The Morality of Abortion: Legal and Historical Perspectives.* Cambridge, Mass.: Harvard Univ. Press, 1970.

*The Oath Book or Red Parchment Book of Colchester.* Trans. and transcribed W. Gurney Benham. Colchester: Essex County, 1907.

*Obstetrics.* Ed. J. P. Greenhill. 13th ed. Philadelphia and London: Saunders, 1965.

Ogg, David. *England in the Reign of Charles II.* 2 vols. 1934, 2nd. ed. 1956; rpt. London: Oxford Univ. Press, 1963.

*Pamphile et Galatée.* Ed. Joseph de Morawski. Paris: Champion, 1917.

Philippe de Navarre. *Les Quatre Ages de l'Homme.* Ed. Marcel de Fréville. Société des Anciens Textes Français. 1888; rpt. New York: Johnson Reprint Corp., 1968.

*Pierce the Ploughmans Crede.* Ed. W. W. Skeat. Early English Text Soc., 30. London: Trübner, 1867.

*Place Names of Gloucestershire.* Ed. A. H. Smith. English Place-Name Society, 38. Cambridge: Cambridge Univ. Press, 1964.

Pliny. *Naturalis Historiae Libri.* XXXVII. Ed. C. Mayhoff. 5 vols. Leipzig: Teubner, 1892–1909.

Power, Eileen. "The Position of Women." *The Legacy of the Middle Ages.* Ed. Charles George Crump and E. F. Jacob. 1926; rpt. Oxford: Clarendon Press, 1943.

*Promptorium Parvulorum.* Ed. Albert Way. London: Camden Society, 1843–65.

Rabelais. *Gargantua and Pantagruel.* Trans. Sir Thomas Urquhart and Peter le Motteaux. 3 vols. 1900; rpt. New York: AMS Press, 1967.

Raine, James, ed. *Fabric Rolls of York Minster.* Surtees Society, 35. Durham: George Andrews, 1859.

Regino of Prum. "De Ecclesiasticis Disciplinis." *Patrologia Latina.* Vol. 132. Ed. J. P. Migne. Paris, 1880.

Ricci, James V. *The Genealogy of Gynaecology.* 2nd ed. enlarged and revised. 1943; rpt. Philadelphia: Blackiston, 1950.

Robbins, Rossell Hope. "The Physician's Authorities." In *Studies in Language and Literature in Honour of Margaret Schlauch.* Warsaw: P. W. Naukowe, 1966.

————. "Mirth in Manuscripts." *Essays and Studies*, 21 (1968), 1–28.

————. "Medical Manuscripts in Middle English." *Speculum*, 45 (1970), 393–415.

————. "Signs of Death in Middle English." *Mediaeval Studies*, 32 (1970), 282–98.

————. "A Note on the Singer Survey of Medical Manuscripts in the British Isles." *Chaucer Review*, 4 (1970), 66–70.

Roberti, Francesco, comp. *Dictionary of Moral Theology.* Westminster, Md.: Newman, 1962.

Roger de Baron. *Practica.* Venice, 1513.

*Le Roman de la Rose.* Ed. Ernest Langlois. 5 vols. Paris: Firmin Didot, 1914–24.

Rösslin, Eucharius. *Eucharius Rösslin's Rosengarten* [Der Swangern Frawen und Hebammen Rosegarten. 1513]. Ed. Gustav Klein. Munich: C. Kuhn, 1910.

Rowland, Beryl. "Exhuming Trotula, *Sapiens Matrona* of Salerno." *Florilegium,* 1 (1979), 42–57.

Ruiz, Juan. *Arcipreste de Hita, Libro de Buen Amor.* Ed. J. C. Y. Frauca. 2 vols. Madrid: Espasa-Calpe, 1960.

Sarton, George. *Introduction to the History of Science.* 3 vols. Baltimore: Williams & Wilkins, 1927–48.

Savonarola, M. *Practica Major.* Colle: 1478.

Scott, Sir Walter. *Letters on Demonology and Witchcraft.* Introd. R. L. Brown. New York: Citadel Press, 1970.

Sigerist, Henry E. "Bedside Manners in the Middle Ages: 'De Cautelis Medicorum,' attributed to Arnold of Villanova." *Quarterly Bulletin of Northwestern University Medical School,* 20 (1946), 136–43.

Singer, Charles, ed. *Studies in the History and Method of Science.* 2 vols. Oxford: Clarendon Press, 1917.

——— and Dorothea Singer. "The Origin of the Medical School of Salerno, the First University. An Attempted Reconstruction." In *Essays on the History of Medicine Presented to Karl Sudhoff.* London: Oxford Univ. Press, 1924.

Smellie, W. *A Treatise on the Theory and Practice of Midwifery.* [1752] 3 vols. London: Strahan, 1779.

Soranus. *Gynaeciorum.* Ed. Valentine Rose. Leipzig: Teubner, 1882.

———. *Gynecology.* Trans. Owsei Temkin. Baltimore: Johns Hopkins, 1956.

Speert, Harold. *Iconographia Gyniatrica.* Philadelphia: F. A. Davis, 1973.

Stephens, George. "Observations on an Old English Medical Manuscript" [in Royal Library, Stockholm]. *Archaeologia,* 30 (1844), 416–18.

Strassburg, Gottfried von. *Tristan und Isolt.* Ed. August Cross. Oxford: Blackwell, 1965.

Szwarcberg, R., P. H. Houyet, and B. Keller. "Accrochage de jumeaux: une circonstance obstétricale exceptionnelle." *Revue française de Gynécologie et de'Obstétrique,* 68 (1973), 59–62.

Tacitus. *Cornelii Taciti De Origine et Situ Germanorum.* Ed. J. G. C. Anderson. Oxford: Clarendon Press, 1938.

———. *The Histories.* Trans. Clifford H. Moore. *The Annals.* Trans. John Jackson. Loeb ed. 4 vols. London: Heinemann, 1963.

Talbot, C. H. "A Mediaeval Physician's Vade Mecum." *Journal of the History of Medicine and Allied Sciences,* 16 (1961), 213–33.

———. *Medicine in Medieval England.* London: Oldbourne, 1967.

———. "Dame Trot and her Progeny." *Essays and Studies,* 25 (1972), 1–14.

———— and E. A. Hammond. *The Medical Practitioners in Mediaeval England: A Bibliographical Register*. London: Wellcome, 1965.

Tertullian. *De Anima*. Ed. Jan Hendrik Waszink. Amsterdam: North Holland Pub., 1947.

Theodorus Priscianus. *Gynaecea ad Saluinam*. Basle: Froben, 1532.

Thomas, Keith. *Religion and the Decline of Magic*. New York: Scribner's, 1971.

Thorndike, Lynn. *A History of Magic and Experimental Science*. 8 vols. New York: Macmillan, 1929–58.

Trachtenburg, Joshua. *Jewish Magic and Superstition*. 1939; rpt. Cleveland and New York: Meridian Books, 1961.

Trotula. *The Diseases of Women by Trotula of Salerno*. Trans. Elizabeth Mason-Hohl. Los Angeles: Ward Ritchie Press, 1940.

Tuttle, Edward F. "The *Trotula* and Old Dame Trot: A Note on the Lady of Salerno." *Bulletin of the History of Medicine*, 50 (1976), 61–72.

Venantius Fortunatus. "Vita Sanctae Radegundis." *Monumenta Germania Historica*. Auctorum Antiquissimorum, IV. 1885; new ed. Berlin: Weidmann, 1961.

Vincent de Beauvais. *Speculum Quadruplex, sive Speculum Maius*. 1624; rpt. of Douai edition. Graz: Akademische Druck, 1964.

Waddams, Herbert. "Abortion." *Dictionary of Christian Ethics*. Ed. John MacQuarrie. Philadelphia: Westminster Press, 1967.

Ward, Bernard. *St. Edmund, Archbishop of Canterbury: His Life As Told by Old English Writers*. London: Sands, 1903.

Wickersheimer, Ernest. *Commentaires de la Faculté de Médecine de l'université de Paris (1395–1516)*. 2 vols. Paris: Imprimerie Nationale, 1915.

————. *Dictionnaire biographique des Médecins en France au moyen âge*. 2 vols. Paris: Librairie E. Droz, 1936.

Williams, George H. "Religious Residues and Presumptions in the American Debate on Abortion." *Theol. Stud.*, 31 (1970), 26–28.

Wolff, Caspar (also known as Hans Kaspar Wolf). *Gynaeciorum*. Basle: T. Guardinus, 1566 [includes *Fragmenta Albucasis*].

Wright, Thomas. *Womankind in Western Europe from the Earliest Times to the Seventeenth Century*. London: Groombridge, 1869.

# INDEX

BERYL ROWLAND is best known for her work on Chaucer and animal symbolism. She is the editor of *Companion to Chaucer Studies* (1968) and *Chaucer and Middle English Studies in Honour of Rossell Hope Robbins* (1974) and the author of *Blind Beasts: Chaucer's Animal World* (1971), *Animals with Human Faces: A Guide to Animal Symbolism* (1974), and *Birds with Human Souls: A Guide to Bird Symbolism* (1978). She has also published many articles, mainly on medieval literature, in professional journals and has lectured extensively at universities in Canada, the United States, Europe, and Australia. She is Professor of English at York University in Toronto and, of particular interest in regard to the present volume, her husband is a physician.